astanga
YOGA

Om, Vande Gurunam Caranaravinde
Sandarsita Svatma Sukhava Bodhe
Nih Sreyase Jangalikayamane
Samsara Halahala Mohasantyai

TRADITIONAL SANSKRIT PRAYER

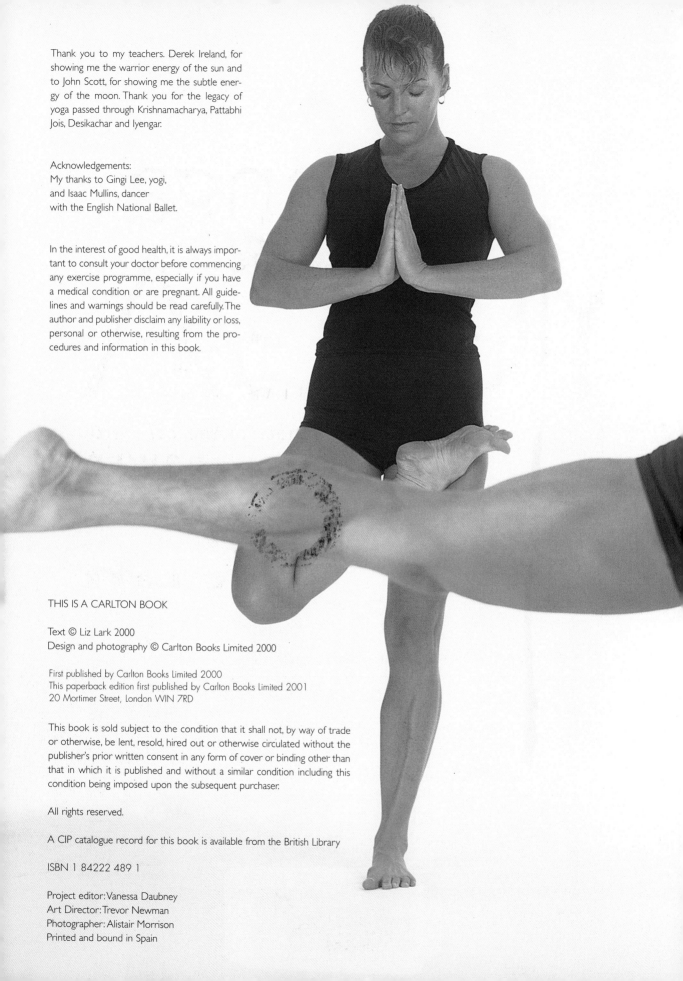

Thank you to my teachers. Derek Ireland, for showing me the warrior energy of the sun and to John Scott, for showing me the subtle energy of the moon. Thank you for the legacy of yoga passed through Krishnamacharya, Pattabhi Jois, Desikachar and Iyengar.

Acknowledgements:
My thanks to Gingi Lee, yogi,
and Isaac Mullins, dancer
with the English National Ballet.

In the interest of good health, it is always important to consult your doctor before commencing any exercise programme, especially if you have a medical condition or are pregnant. All guidelines and warnings should be read carefully. The author and publisher disclaim any liability or loss, personal or otherwise, resulting from the procedures and information in this book.

THIS IS A CARLTON BOOK

Text © Liz Lark 2000
Design and photography © Carlton Books Limited 2000

First published by Carlton Books Limited 2000
This paperback edition first published by Carlton Books Limited 2001
20 Mortimer Street, London WIN 7RD

A CIP catalogue record for this book is available from the British Library

ISBN 1 84222 489 1

Project editor: Vanessa Daubney
Art Director: Trevor Newman
Photographer: Alistair Morrison
Printed and bound in Spain

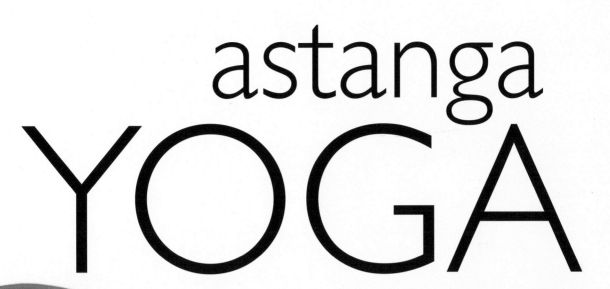

astanga
YOGA

connect to the core with
POWER yoga

Liz Lark

CARLTON
BOOKS

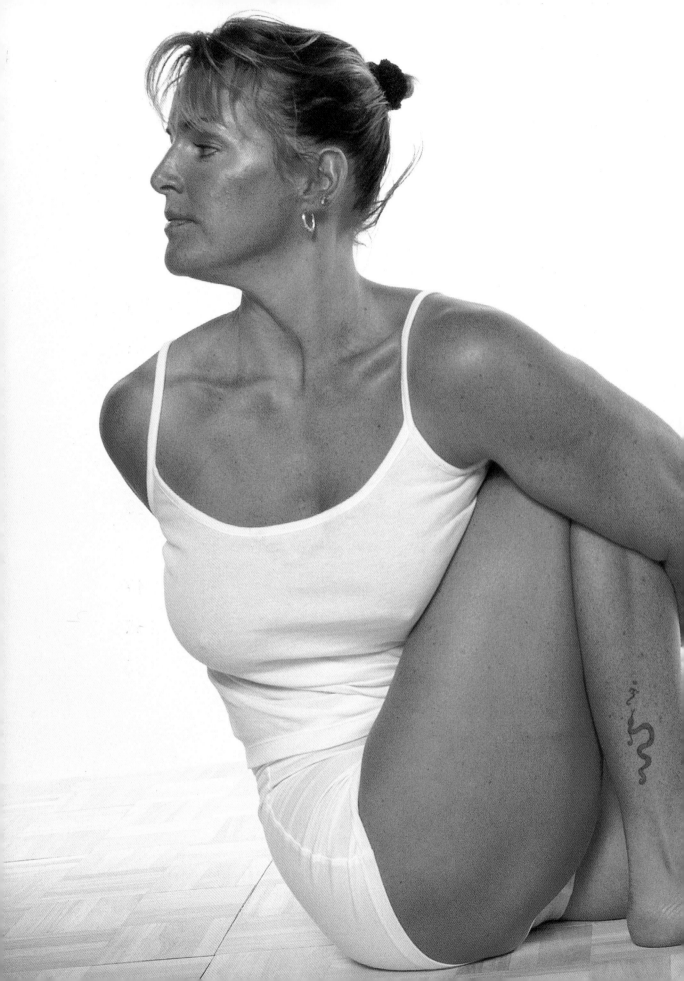

CONTENTS

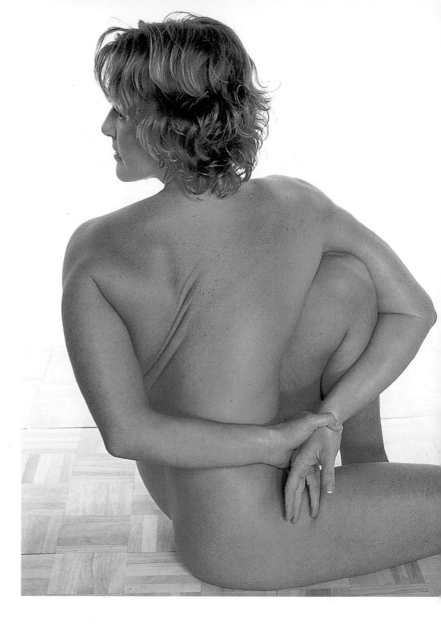

INTRODUCTION

When I left school in 1984 with yuppiedom staring me in the face, I secured my place at Art College, packed my bag and went to the foothills of the Pakistani Himalayas to teach in a hill station school. An antithesis to the material world, I heaved a huge sigh of relief as living in the mountains very simply, I realized that there are other ways of being and other realities. The door to the East had opened and it was like smelling a jasmine flower.

During this time, I visited an ashram in Puna, Maharashtra, in India, where yogis were practising their art and Catholic nuns were studying Hindu, Buddhist and Christian mystic texts and their open spirituality really impressed me and started me thinking.

Then, in 1991, while I was in search of a holiday with a difference, I discovered Astanga yoga in a remote bay in Southern Crete. The Practice Place was the only centre in Europe teaching this rigorous, exhilarating form of yoga and, although I had been practising other forms of softer yoga which Astanga used in its flowing sequence, I was awestruck. I returned every year, leading art and life-drawing workshops and learning the Primary, Intermediate, and some Advanced, series with my teacher Derek Ireland.

As an artist, I evolved from manipulating clay to manipulating bodies and in 1995 I began to teach yoga myself. I was seeking a non-dogmatic, spiritual and creative method which was rooted in nature and which celebrated rather than denied the body. I felt I had found my chosen discipline and form of self-expression in the dance of Astanga, following the thread of the breath.

This book is an introduction to Astanga Vinyasa yoga and presents the Primary Series in its complete form. In the following pages, you will find out a little about what yoga is, where it comes from and what distinguishes Astanga Vinyasa yoga from other forms, such as Hatha yoga, and makes it such a complete psycho-physical form of training. If anything sparks your curiosity, you may like to consult the Bibliography at the end of this book to get some idea of what to read next.

Chapter 3 – The Elements of the Practice – outlines the basics of Astanga yoga, explaining how to build the foundations which will support and strengthen your body and focus your mind. Please read this chapter before you embark on anything else in the book.

The next three chapters take you step-by-step through the Primary Series of Astanga yoga – from the basic sequences called Suryanamaskars via the Standing Postures to the Seated Postures and the Finishing Postures, which close down one's practice and help one move towards relaxation. Build your practice on these three chapters and only move on when you are thoroughly familar and comfortable with the initial poses.

The practice of yoga is not just a form of physical exercise and in Chapters 7 and 8 you will find techniques for relaxation as well as an explanation of the eastern philosophy which concerns the subtle "energy body" that is believed to exist within the physical body.

I would like to stress, though, that this book is not a complete substitute for a good, qualified teacher and it should really be used to accompany and encourage you as you embark on a course, particularly when it comes to the more advanced poses. Hopefully, it will help to clarify the postures and act to jog your memory when you practise by yourself. Above all, be kind to yourself, this is not some kind of army physical training course, although it has been referred to as hippy meets army bootcamp! It is an ancient system of artful sculpting, challenging the body to unlock. Listen to your body and what it tells you as you practise. Work to your edge, that is, the limit you are capable of achieving, and follow the thread of the breath.

You are a piece of calligraphy. Write yourself.

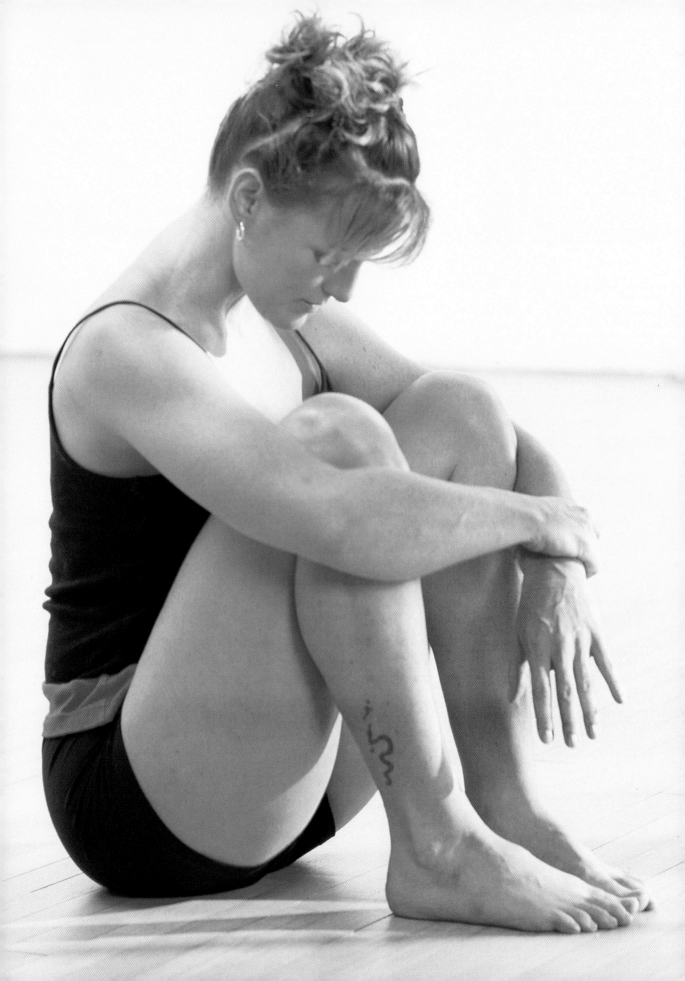

I

CONNECT TO
THE CORE WHAT IS YOGA?

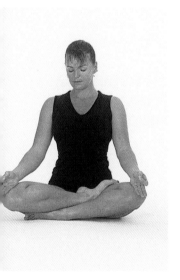

The practice of yoga dates back over five thousand years to the time of ancient forest dwellers called "Rishis", sages who dwelt in the Indus Valley, in what is now northern India. Observing nature and searching within themselves, they evolved physical postures and breathing exercises which stretched, cleansed and centred the body, cultivating states of vitality, clarity and focus.

Yoga means "union": to yolk, or unite, and comes from the Sanskrit root *yuj*.

Through the practice of yoga, we are aiming to integrate the body, mind and emotions to bring about a state of balance, drawing ourselves deeper into the present in search of the eternal moment.

There are many different forms of yoga providing numerous pathways from which we can choose. They include:

HATHA YOGA – SUN (HA) – MOON (THA) UNION

This union is achieved through psychophysical (mind/body) training, which balances the sun principle *(yang)* – the active, dynamic, masculine aspects of ourselves – with the moon principle *(yin)* – our intuitive, sensitive, feminine aspects.

KARMA YOGA

Karma means action and Karma yoga concerns a balance or union through selfless action or service. This form of yoga is best suited to those with vigorous temperaments who feel called to serve in human affairs.

BHAKTI YOGA

Bhakti means emotional devotion felt for the 'divine' and is expressed through prayer or worship. The quality of bhakti is found in the world's major religions where the individual self (the ego) reaches out for the greater, universal self (the soul). In this form the yogic (balanced) state is achieved through devotion, love and surrender.

JNANA YOGA

Jnana means knowledge, or intellectual discrimination. It calls for clarity of mind and a rejection of all that is transient or superficial. Jnana yoga achieves union through constant discrimination between what is real and what is unreal, in order to "pierce the veil" between illusion *(maya)* and reality – to see beyond.

RAJA YOGA

Raja yoga combines all forms of yoga and can involve Karma, Jnana and Bhakti. Raja means the yoga of kings and is concerned with the study of the body as a vehicle of spiritual energy. Contemplative in nature, this form is primarily for those called to monastic life. It is the way of meditation, transcending the mind by conscious will.

TANTRA YOGA

This system works with the symbolic *shakti* (or female power) to awaken *kundalini* energy which lies sleeping at the base of the spine (see Chapter 8). Tantra is a combination of all the above-mentioned paths of yoga, using the body as the vehicle to awaken consciousness.

The aim of each form is UNITY of being, achieving a balanced mind by natural methods.

The most practised form of yoga in the West is Hatha yoga, for it gives us a tangible system of physical culture, training the body, breath and mind towards a "one-pointedness" or single focus. Hatha yoga gives us a superb total physical training system of realignment and health, and Astanga Vinyasa yoga is a particularly flowing, dynamic form of Hatha yoga.

ASTANGA VINYASA YOGA – DANCE ON THE BREATH

The beauty of Astanga Vinyasa yoga is its flowing, dance-like sequences, held together on the thread of the breath.

The authentic name for this

Citta vritti nirodhah.
(To still the thought waves of the mind.)

PATANJALI, YOGA SUTRA NO. 2

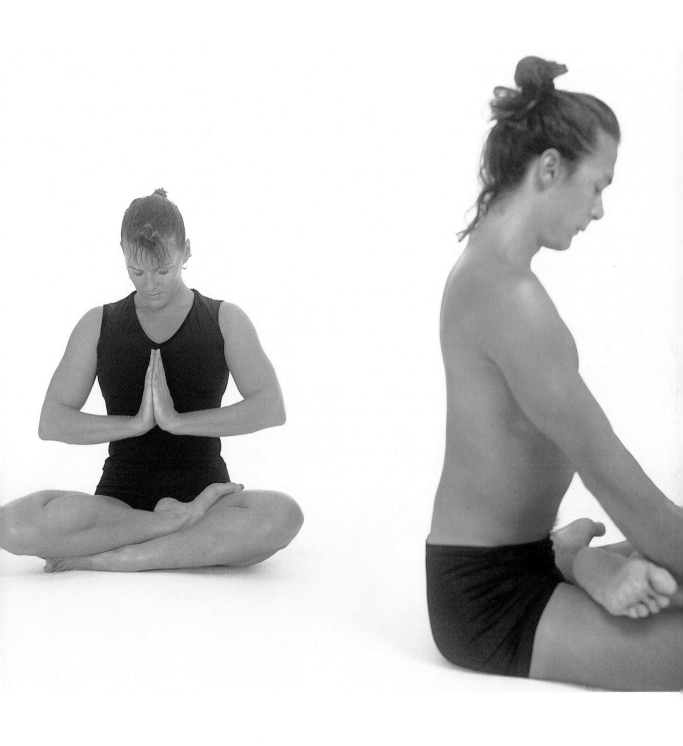

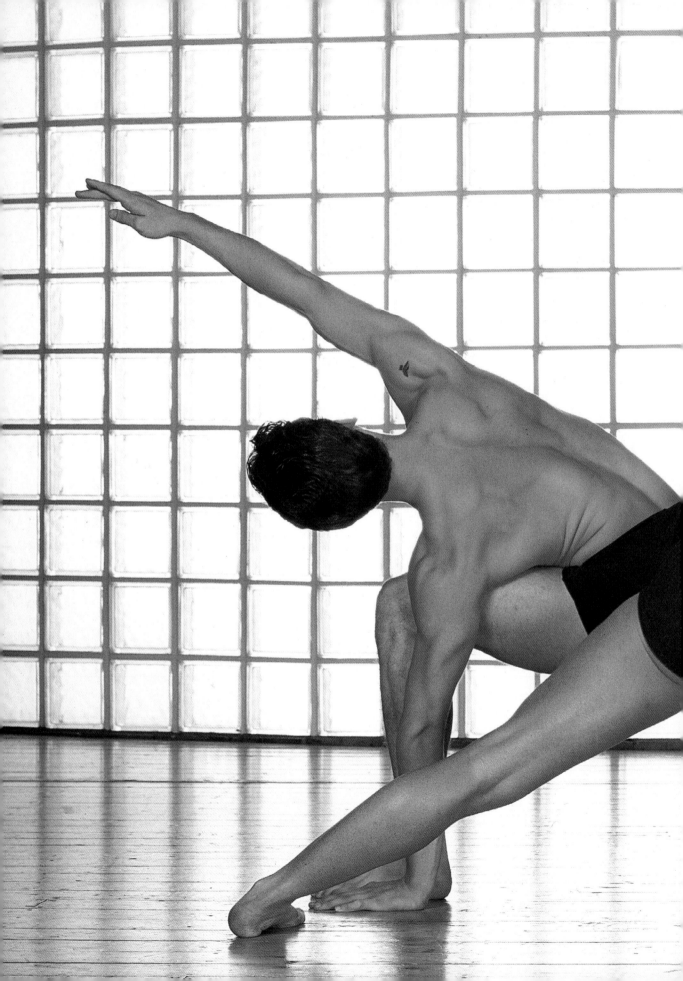

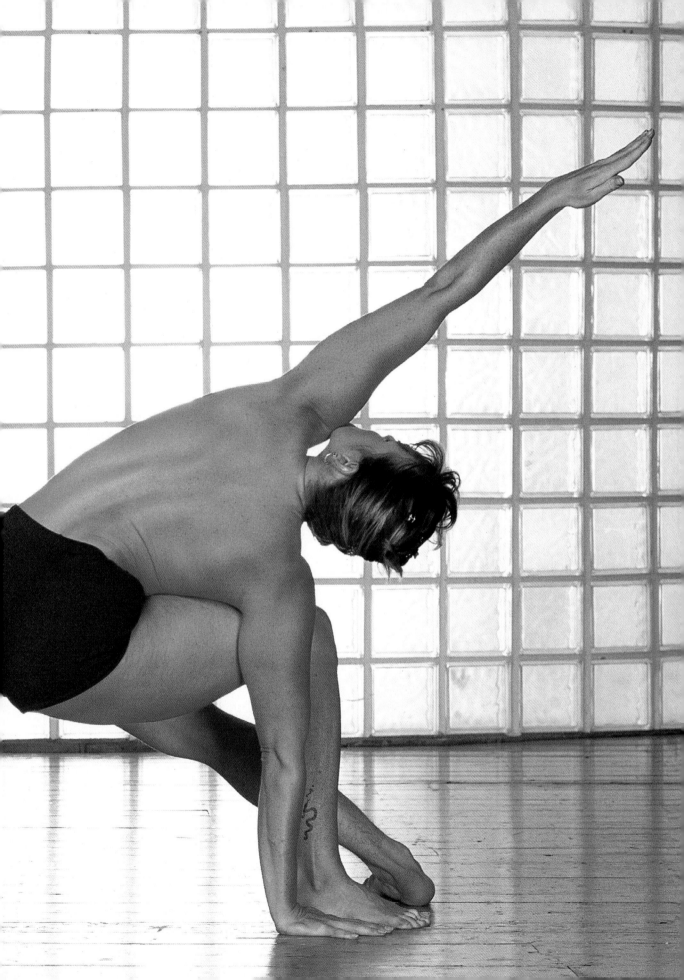

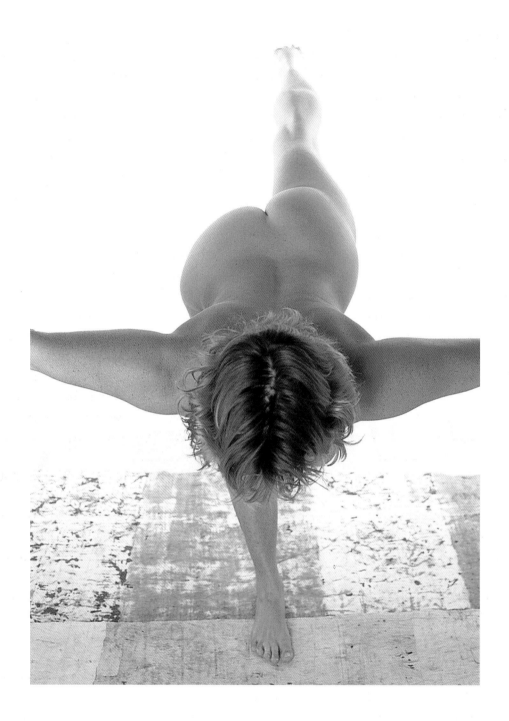

form of yoga is Astanga Vinyasa, though it is currently widely publicized as Power yoga because of its energizing nature and the high level of fitness which comes from practising it.

Astanga yoga is far more than a workout. It is an art, creating a new relationship with the body.

The rigorous discipline of the system gradually leads to mastery over all areas of one's life. The practice is empowering and liberating as emotional and physical blockages are shifted within oneself, moving through fear in a gently unfolding journey towards self-acceptance. Through meditation in movement, the deeper purpose is to still the mind and open the heart.

Body postures (*asanas*) are synchronized with a controlled breathing system (*ujjayi pranayama*) held together with inner energy body locks (*bandhas*) in a choreographed sequence. Constant, controlled activity is combined with a heightened energy level, toning the body into maximum fitness and giving it balance.

The basic practice is designed to realign the body therapeutically, freeing the muscular system and rebalancing the skeletal system. Through it the spine is reawakened and made lithe, yet also (as yogic texts describe) as "strong as a thunderbolt".

Body postures are linked together by *vinyasas* (breath-synchronized movements) which create a deep, purifying heat, nourishing internal organs and eliminating toxins.

The nervous system is soothed and the blood purified, while internal cleansing takes place through the alchemy of breath and movement, releasing power and energy which can be exhilarating.

Physiologically, a complete fitness system, a remarkable combination of strength, flexibility and stamina follows, opening an exciting pathway to lifelong health, and a deep level of relaxation, which is accompanied by a sense of rejuvenation.

Astanga is *mind-medicine:* the mind is softened and focused as one sheds tensions and disease.

AST-ANGA – THE EIGHT LIMBS OF PATANJALI

Astanga comes from the words *ast*, meaning eight, and *anga,* meaning limbs. Vinyasa means breath-connected movement.

Between 400 BC and AD 400, the sage Patanjali crystallized the components of classical Astanga yoga in *sutras*, meaning threads of wisdom. He prescribed a *sadhana* (path) of eight limbs, in a rigorous disciplined approach to guide the soul towards emancipation, and to release the ties of the material world. The goal was to clear the clouding of the intelligence in order to transform the mind from its scattered state in a sea of chaos to become single-pointed. The sutras he laid down are a practical aid to the spiritual life and have universal significance. They can be interpreted by any individual.

The first four limbs are external, the second four internal. Limbs one to four involve physical effort and the conscious training of the mind and body; while limbs five to eight lead from gross, material practices to subtle, spiritual practices where the deeper recesses of the mind are brought to light and cleansed. Like peeling away the layers of an onion, the journey of yoga becomes a stripping away of the layers of conditioned existence, which leads to self-awareness and self-knowledge.

The external limbs may be seen as a means of taming the ego (or conscious mind) and the internal limbs

as the awakening of the self, or soul. In yoga, the ego needs to be harnessed in order to liberate the soul. The Mundaka Upanishad* beautifully describes the dichotomy of the higher and lower self residing in the body: "Like two birds on the selfsame tree, the ego and the soul sit side by side in the body. The former stares about him, pecking at the sweet fruit, indulges and tastes the fruits of life whilst the latter watches, discriminating."

The insatiable appetite of the ego is never satisfied and the passage goes on to explain: "The personal self, weary of pecking here and there sinks into dejection; but when it understands through meditation that the other, the impersonal self is indeed spirit, dejection disappears."

THE EXTERNAL LIMBS
1. YAMA – ETHICS

This is the basis of moral behaviour and covers one's attitudes towards the environment. Yama consists of five sub-limbs: *Ahimsa* (non-violence), *Satya* (truthfulness), *Asteya* (non-stealing), *Brahmacharya* (continence, containing the vital essence of controlling sexual energy), and *Aparigraha* (non-possessiveness).

*The Upanishads date from around 600 BC, when Buddha was born. They contain the oldest philosophical compositions of the world and were passed on aurally, sung by forest sages, long before they were written down. Upanishads literally mean "at the feet of...[some master]".

2. NIYAMA – SELF-DISCIPLINE

This limb involves our attitude towards ourselves and also consists of five sub-limbs: *Saucha* (inner and outer body purification), *Santosha* (contentment), *Tapas* (discipline), *Swadhyaya* (study of spiritual books), and *Ishwara Pranadhanini* (surrender – *Ishwara* means the lord of nature).

3. ASANA – THE PRACTICE OF BODILY POSTURES

This is the first conscious step on the path of yoga, cleaning the vessel of the body, the aim being to build a strong, healthy body, which has a direct impact on the mind.

4. PRANAYAMA – THE SCIENCE OF BREATHING

A system of breathing techniques for cleansing the body, which thereby calms and concentrates the mind.

THE INTERNAL LIMBS

5. PRATYAHARA – WITHDRAWAL OF THE SENSES

Through this practice one can loosen the grip of the ties which bind us, i.e. habits, or addictions. It is where the journey from the outer world of the ego to the inner world of the soul begins. (Pranayama and Pratyahara develop tranquillity.)

6. DHARANA – CONCENTRATION

The ability to direct the mind, to hold it in a single line of focus, uninterrupted.

7. DHYANA – MEDITATION

The process by which one connects with that which one seeks to understand, by concentrating the mind on the object of focus. (Dharana and Dhyana prepare the soul for Samadhi.)

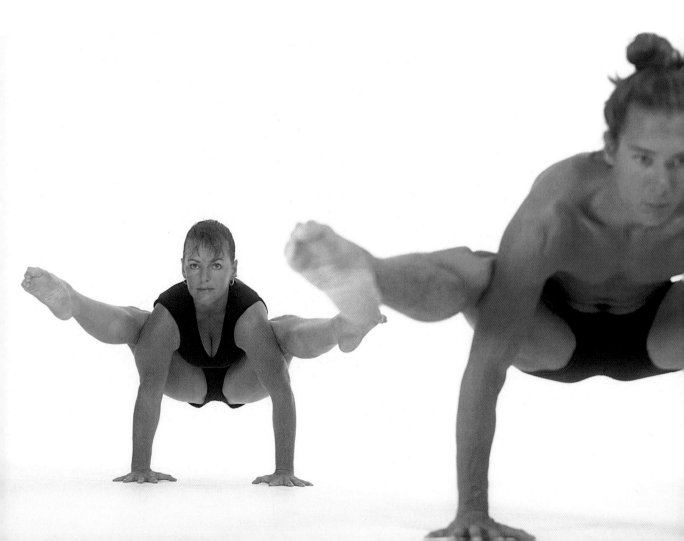

8. SAMADHI – ABSORPTION

The final limb is where the practitioner of yoga has reached a state of integration and transcendence, when the creative mind is immersed in a pool of bliss. It is in essence the achievement of mind mastery.

Self rides in the chariot of the body, intellect the firm-rooted charioteer, discursive mind the reins. Senses are the horses, objects of desire the roads. When self is joined to body, mind, sense, none but He enjoys.

When a (wo)man lacks steadiness, unable to control his mind, his senses are unmanageable horses. But if he control his mind, a steady man, they are manageable horses.

Book I, Katha Upanishad

Patanjali describes the mind as a chariot pulled by wild horses, which toss it this way and that. The eight limbs of yoga offer a system to tame the wild horses of the mind, learning to drive the vehicle of the body. We build the foundation of this training with asana (posture) and pranayama (breathing practice).

It is very difficult to practise the first two limbs of yoga, says Sri K. Pattabhi Jois, the master teacher of Astanga Vinyasa, if we have a weak body and a weak mind, so we strengthen the body with limbs three and four.

In the practice of Astanga, we endeavour to integrate all limbs. Extending the breath through the asana, we withdraw the senses (pratyahara) from the outer world by concentrating (dharana) on the practice. The practice becomes a moving meditation (dhyana) on the sound of the breath (pranayama) in a seamless sequence, bringing about a state of absorption (samadhi).

If the mind folds itself to a point of concentration or becomes standstill, as it were, it can keep the body and the senses under its control, so that there will not be a possibility of their getting diseases. If the mind becomes weak, it will be the cause of many diseases, hallucinations and other mental distortions which give rise to physical diseases. The process of disciplining and purifying the mind is called yoga.

SRI K. PATTABHI JOIS

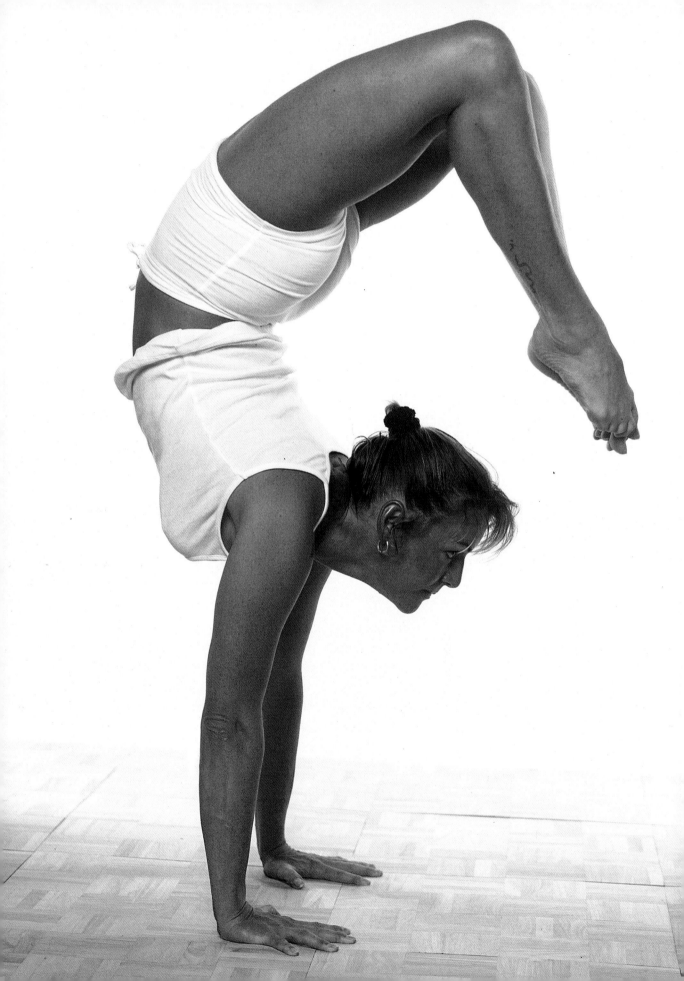

2

THE DISCOVERY OF THE YOGA KORUNTA

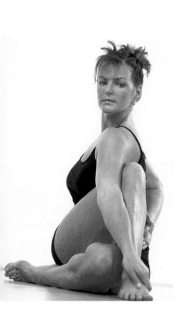

In the early 1930s, Sri Krishnamacharya, an accomplished scholar and yogi, was perusing texts in the University of Calcutta's library with his student, Sri K. Pattabhi Jois. The story goes that the master teacher stumbled across a body of information written on leaves and bound together as a manuscript, containing a detailed system of yoga, written in Sanskrit by an ancient seer named Vamana Rishi.

The text was estimated to be between five hundred and fifteen hundred years old, although the Sanskrit verse used was thought to be part of an older oral tradition, which dates back as much as five thousand years.

The documents consisted of hundreds of detailed rhyming stanzas, describing an intricate system of how to enter and exit asanas, breathing techniques and linking movements, applications and benefits.

Sri Krishnamacharya deciphered this priceless text, and incorporated the *Yoga Korunta* into his teaching and methodology. But it was Sri K. Pattabhi Jois who became the principal teacher of the form, dedicatedly teaching the pure form of Astanga, which came to be known as the 'Mysore style' and which is now awakening interest across the globe.

THE SERIES – 'FREEDOM THROUGH A FORM'

The distinction between Astanga Vinyasa and other forms of yoga is the vinyasa, a continuous, dynamic flow, linking breath and movement, and its detailed specific structure and order of postures. Vamana Rishi, the author of the *Yoga Korunta*, is believed to have said: "Oh yogi, don't do asana without vinyasa."

There are three "series", or sequences, within the Astanga yoga system, each consisting of approximately forty postures and lasting between one and a half and two hours.

The first, or "primary series", is called *Yoga Chikitsa*, meaning yoga therapy, which realigns the spine and detoxifies the body, building a foundation of considerable physical strength, flexibility and stamina. It is a complete system which, if followed step by step, works like a combination lock, artfully opening up the body. Each series unlocks a particular aspect of the body and mind and when the series is learnt, one can practise on a more subconscious level, in an unbroken flowing sequence. The primary series is a gift for a lifetime, becoming deeper with regular practice.

Pattabhi Jois says: "To practise a long time with respect and without interruption brings perfection. One, two years, ten years... your entire life long, you practise."

If you practise the opening sequence with presence of mind, correct breathing and deep focus, you can receive the gift of yoga: namely balance, integration, and union.

Even after one session the body feels energized, the eyes are clear and the mind is calm. But the yoga is not a quick fix. Regular practice is necessary, though don't worry if you can't master every posture. It takes time. Once the primary series is correctly practised, the intermediate series, *Nadi Shodana*, meaning nerve purification, is introduced by the teacher. The practice cleanses the *nadis*, or subtle nerve channels, in the body (see Chapter 8), and purifies and strengthens the nervous system. The spine is made lithe and strong like a plant stem through a sequence of back bends; hips and hamstrings are eased open and the upper body is developed further with arm balances, and steadiness is cultivated in a series of headstands.

The advanced series is subdivided into four sections collectively called *Sthira Bhaga*, which is translated as "divine stability". *Sthira* means steadiness, or strength, and *Bhaga* means good fortune, dignity, beauty. Considerable endurance, control and humility are required and very few aspirants practise this awe-inspiring sequence.

KRISHNAMACHARYA – A TWENTIETH-CENTURY MASTER TEACHER

Sri Tirumalai Krishnamacharya was renowned in India as an authority on Indian philosophy, Sanskrit literature, religion, music and Ayurveda (southern Indian traditional medicine). He helped to revive and popularize Hatha yoga in India, and the form he evolved spread internationally via his students T. K. V. Desikachar (his son, who has specialized in Viniyoga, or yoga therapy), B. K. S. Iyengar (master of asana, precision and depth of alignment) and Sri K. Pattabhi Jois (master of Astanga Vinyasa yoga). All three teachers, who are now in their eighties, continue their work today in Madras, Pune and Mysore respec-

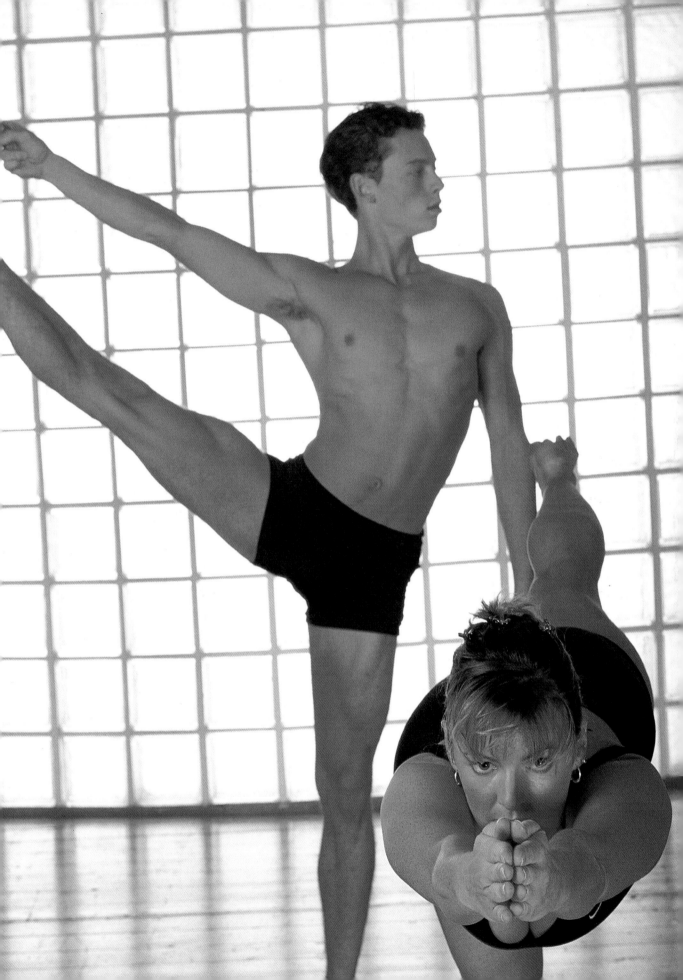

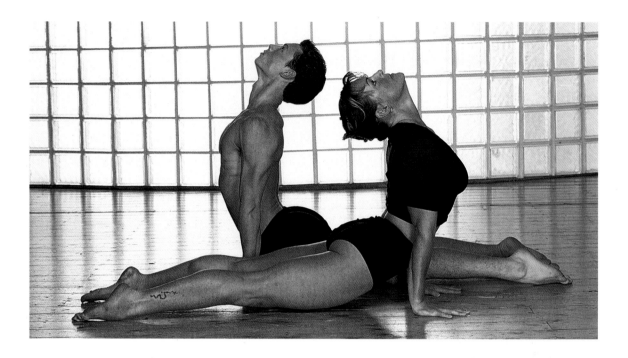

tively, and their methods are spreading throughout the world.

Krishnamacharya was born in 1891 into a family of yoga teachers that can trace its ancestry back to Nathamundi, a ninth-century Indian sage. In his early life, Krishnamacharya travelled all over India and Tibet learning religious practices, in search of authentic Hatha yoga, and in 1919, at the age of twenty-seven, he found his teacher in a cave in Tibet. At first, Sri Ramamohan Brahnachari, a father of eight children, who lived to be one hundred and fifty, refused to teach Krishnamacharya. So for eight days Krishnamacharya refused to eat, until Ramamohan gave him two chapatis to send him away! But still, he would not leave; finally they conversed in Sanskrit and Krishnamacharya remained there for seven years.

Thus, Krishnamacharya was strongly influenced by Tibetan Buddhist yoga. He learnt vinyasa and the jumping style of practice, which he later discovered in the *Yoga Korunta*, and for which B. K. S. Iyengar and Pattabhi Jois have since become renowned.

In 1930, the Maharaja of Mysore became his student, and in 1934, Krishnamacharya was invited to head the yogashala (yoga house) in the palace. The building now houses the art collection. Krishnamacharya remained at the palace yogashala for twenty years.

A radical pioneer who rejected labels and was known to challenge dogmatic beliefs, Krishnamacharya was one of the first to dispute the idea that yoga and vedic chanting should not be taught to women or outcastes. He received the equivalent of masters and Ph.D degrees, memorizing entire writings of Hindu, Jain and Buddhist philosophical texts and was not only a scholar, but also an adept yogi who was able to stop the beating of his heart. Tested by several doctors, they surmised that Krishnamacharya had decreased the venous bloodflow back to the heart to such an extent that it was not possible to detect a pulse for more than two minutes. Still teaching at ninety-six, Krishnamacharya died at the age of one hundred in Madras, in 1989, leaving a rich, spiritual legacy.

GURU SRI K. PATTABHI JOIS

Born in 1915 in Mysore, in southern India, Sri K. Pattabhi Jois met Krishnamacharya when he was twelve years old, and studied under him from 1927 to 1945. He first learnt asana and pranayama, the foundations of yoga, and later studied Sanskrit and Advaita Vedanta philosophy at the Sanskrit College of Mysore, becoming a professor there, teaching Sanskrit and philosophy, for thirty-six years.

In 1937, Pattabhi Jois began teaching yoga at the Sanskrit College and to the present day he teaches at his yogashala in his home in Mysore with his grandson, Sharat. Pattabhi Jois has made Astanga yoga into a thriving, living system, and has also made it accessible to the West in its undiluted form through his dedication to the pure "Mysore style".

THE GERMINATION OF ASTANGA IN THE WEST

In the 1960s, the first foreign student, a writer and yoga teacher named Andrei Van Lysbeth from Belgium, visited Pattabhi Jois. He had been to India many times, studying with expert teachers including B. K. S. Iyengar and Sivananda. Following Van Lysbeth in the early 1970s, two "twenty-something" spiritual seekers, David Williams and Norman Allen, were travelling in India, staying in an ashram in Pondicherry. Pattabhi Jois's son, Manju, was giving an Astanga demonstration in the ashram, which inspired the two Americans and, just as Krishnamacharya had waited on the steps of his teacher's home in Tibet, so Norman Allen begged for instruction outside Pattabhi Jois's yogashala, but Pattabhi Jois refused to teach him.

Eventually, Pattabhi Jois relented, and Allen spent two years in Mysore learning the yoga and earning a masters degree in Indian studies.

David Williams and another student, Nancy Gilgoff, also studied under Pattabhi Jois, and Williams became the first westerner to master the whole series.

In keeping with 1970s counterculture, Williams and Nancy Gilgoff established their school on Maui, in a studio donated by a grateful practitioner who claims that Astanga yoga saved his life. The humid Hawaiian climate and relaxed culture provided an ideal Petri dish in which to grow Astanga, which then developed in California.

In recent years, Astanga has gradually become established in the West and is now flourishing, having come a long way from the yogashala of Sri K. Pattabhi Jois in Mysore.

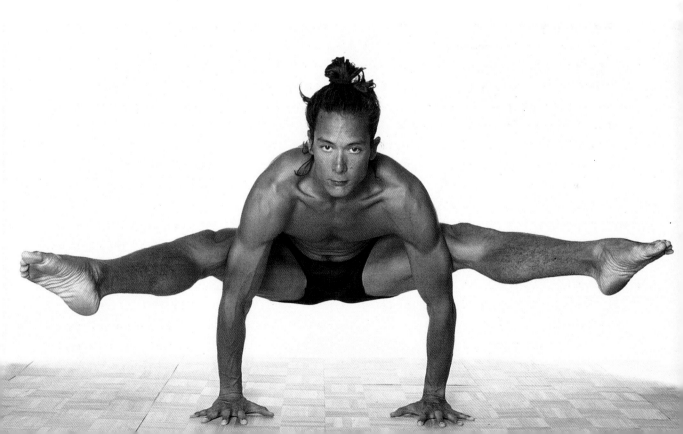

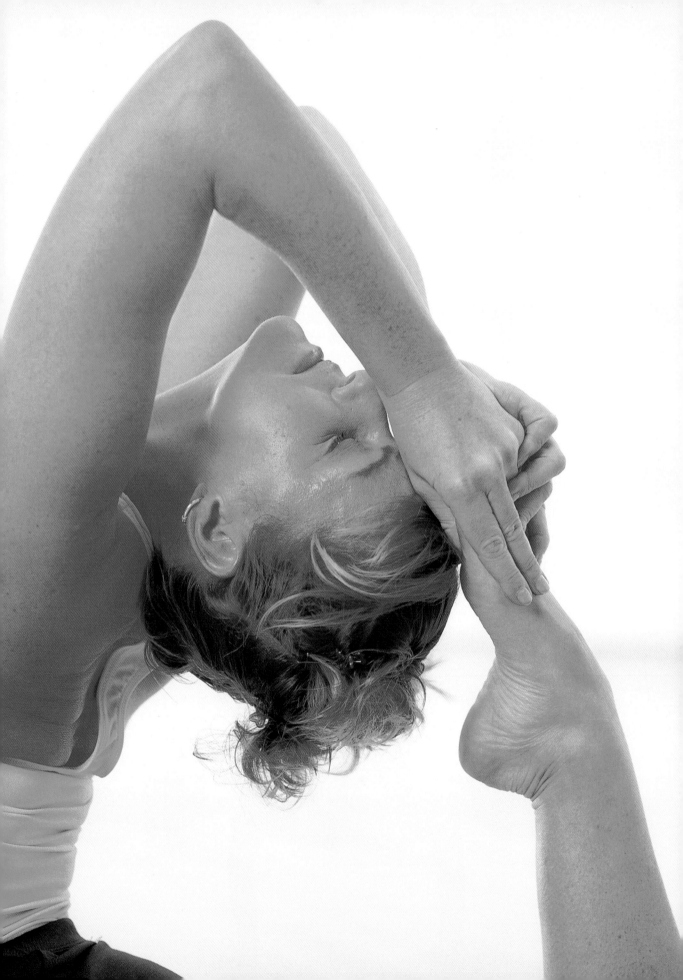

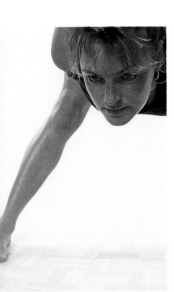

3

THE ELEMENTS OF THE PRACTICE

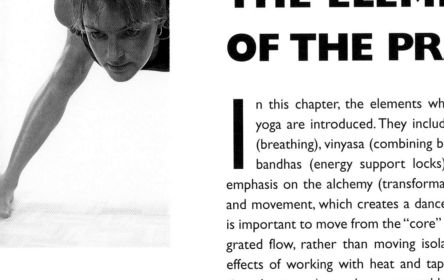

In this chapter, the elements which form the basis of Astanga yoga are introduced. They include asanas (posture), pranayama (breathing), vinyasa (combining breath with movement) and the bandhas (energy support locks). Astanga Vinyasa yoga places emphasis on the alchemy (transformation) brought about by breath and movement, which creates a dance of tapas (intense discipline).It is important to move from the "core" (centre) of the body in an integrated flow, rather than moving isolated body parts. The cleansing effects of working with heat and tapas, so lifting *samskaras* (conditioned patterns), are also presented here, revealing the deeper mental and emotional benefits which come with the practice of yoga as one sheds "the poison of conditioned existence".

This book is a visual support to accompany your practice. First, find a teacher, or go on an intensive course to learn the foundations safely. Then, practise, and return to classes as often as you can. Although practising by yourself will bring about enormous benefits, having access to a teacher will help you to correct your alignment and make sure that you are moving into postures correctly. But, like learning to swim, the real journey begins when you go out into the ocean by yourself.

Make the yoga your own, learn from the inside, noticing any sensations in your body as you practise. We are aiming to awaken the intelligence of the body. So, above all else, keep practising and listen to your body and breathing.

CORE STRENGTH

In yoga, movement is initiated from the inside, or the core of the body. We move from the pelvis and the spine, i.e. from the bones and the central structure of the body, rather than from outer muscle strength. Yogic postures stretch, lengthen and tone muscles rather than contracting and tightening them.

SPEAKING DIRECTLY TO THE BODY

Instructions are given directly to different body parts and it is important to direct the mind into the body, to awaken the body's innate intelligence and move from the bones and the deep inner muscles instinctively.

Phrases such as "open", "lengthen", "create space", "release" and "surrender" are terms to engender internal awareness of the body, and of stretching without strain or tension. We approach the movement in a creative, flowing sense rather than a defined, set, linear sense.

The word "pelvis" means basin and it is the pelvis which receives the weight of the upper body and passes the weight to the lower limbs. The pelvis absorbs the stresses of the lower limbs, and the pelvic floor, which consists of a cluster of nerves and muscles, is the floor of the torso – the base support, just as our feet support our bodies.

THE SUPPORT OF THE BANDHAS

We create core strength by harnessing inner body locks called bandhas, which mean "grips". Think of the pelvis like a garden, containing nutrients and soil. Support this garden by walling it; the front wall of the lower abdomen is sealed inwards with the deep muscle band contraction of Uddiyana bandha (see page 30), which goes from hip bone to hip bone, and relates to the corset-like transverse muscle that runs round the abdomen. The front wall of the garden is sealed towards the back wall, or the sacrum, the wedge-shaped component of the pelvic basin.

We support the floor of the pelvis, and of the whole trunk of the body, by lifting the cluster of muscles of the perineum, which is between the

anus and the genitals. This is the Mula bandha (see page 30) or root lock.

From the garden of the pelvic basin, which is made secure and strong with the two lower locks (bandhas) we grow the spine upwards, out of the pelvis, like a plant stem.

Through the yoga asanas, the spine becomes sanguine, lithe yet strong, felt by the rising energy from the pelvic garden, resisting the gravitational pull. The top of the spine lifts the base of the skull and the crown of the head, the closest point to heaven, is drawn upwards.

This sense of moving from the core, the centre, i.e. the pelvis and spine, and *hara*, the belly (known in the East as the seat of the soul, which is why such phrases as "gut reaction" make sense to us), supported by core strength, creates a strong, centred body. This helps to bring about a balance of the left and right sides of the body.

Anyone who has had experience of such forms of complementary bodywork as the Alexander Technique or the "release" techniques of new dance and physical theatre will know how they help to cultivate awareness of moving instinctively from the deep centre of the body.

ASANA

Asana means to sit, or rest, and comes from the root *as*, which means to sit. Asana, or posture, is the first conscious step on the path of yoga, creating a strong, healthy,

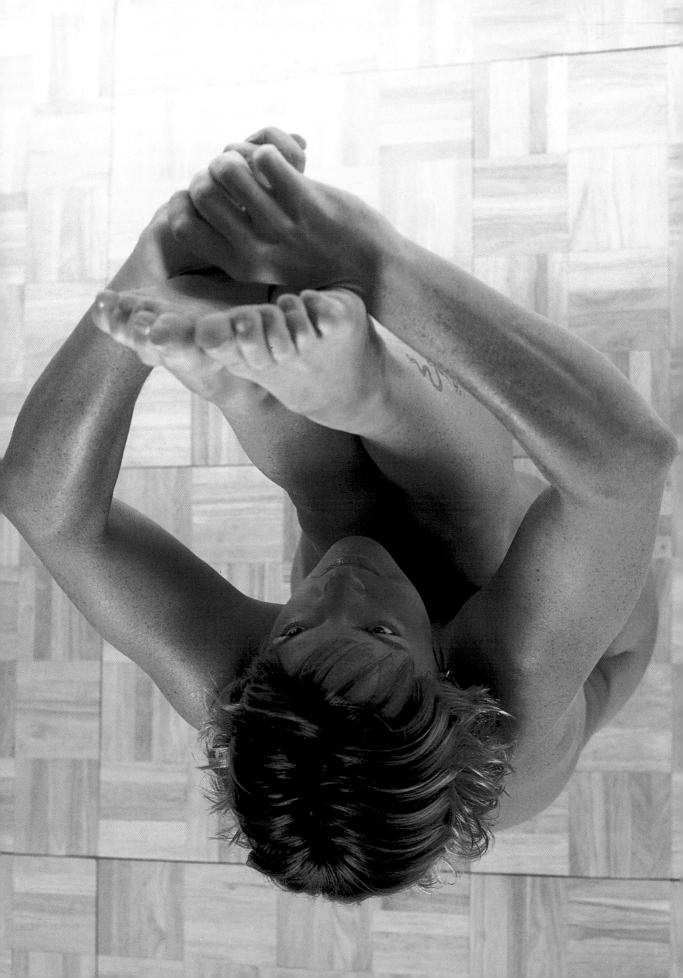

detoxified body. Asanas provide the means for building up willpower to transcend physical and mental boundaries by determination, cultivating physical and psychological strength.

PRANAYAMA (BREATHING) – THE HEART OF THE PRACTICE

Pranayama is the art of controlling the breath. *Prana* means that which is infinitely everywhere, while *Ayama* means to stretch, or extend.

For centuries, meditators have regulated the breath in order to soothe the mind. Deep, conscious breathing strengthens the lungs, nourishes the body, soothes and steadies the mind, creating a feeling of internal space. The Ancients taught that we have been given a set number of breaths (21,600 per day) and one hundred years to live. Slow conscious breathing can increase a lifespan up to one hundred and fifty years.

The breath is the guiding force of the practice of Astanga yoga. We use it to support our movements and oscillate muscles and joints, thus awakening the intelligence of the body. The breath diffuses energy through the body like the waves of the sea. This energy is called prana.

The inhalation (*puraka*) is the cleansing wave, which increases prana; and the exhalation (*rechaka*) is the detox wave, eliminating impurities and making room for more prana to enter. The aim of conscious breathing (pranayama) is to balance the inhalation with the exhalation. This draws the mind's focus inwards, channelling thoughts within, and facilitating meditation while in motion.

When a person is lacking in prana, he or she has the feeling of being stuck or restricted, and has a lack of drive. It is no surprise therefore that we may feel depleted of energy in the cities, for prana is cultivated with fresh air and vital, *sattwic* (pure, fresh) foods.

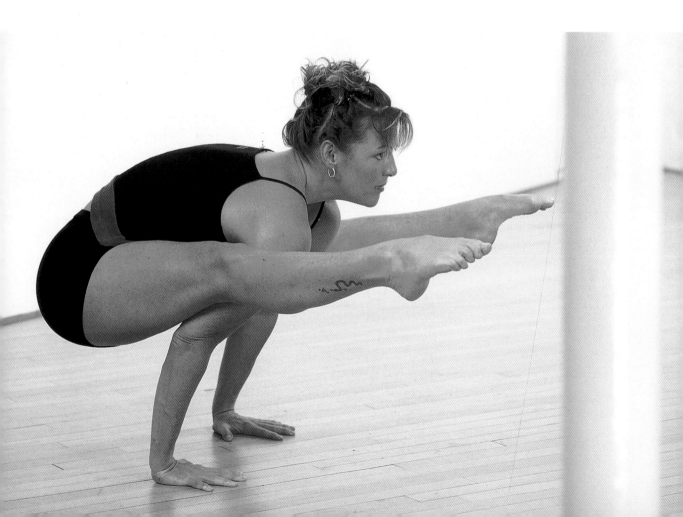

Your pain is the breaking of the shell that encloses your understanding. Much of your pain is self-chosen. It is the bitter potion by which the physician within you heals your sick self.

KAHLIL GIBRAN, 'THE PROPHET'

UJJAYI BREATH – VICTORIOUS STRETCHING OF THE INNER BREATH

Ujjayi comes from *Ud*, meaning extreme, and *Jayi*, meaning to conquer, or subdue. *Ujjayi* means "victorious stretching of the inner breath".

Throughout the Astanga practice, we breathe the Ujjayi breath, a thoracic, chest breath, which brings conscious awareness to the expansion of the ribcage, drawing fresh prana into the body and creating internal heat.

The breath, combined with the stretching movements (vinyasas), cleanses the nervous and circulatory systems with discipline and sweat.

METHOD:

Gently narrow the glottis at the back of the throat, squeezing it like a valve, to channel the breath back and forth through the roof of the palette, deep into the lungs.

The breathing is now a deep, thoracic, chest breath, centred in the ribcage. It feels as if you are about to yawn, but don't open your mouth. Soften the face and jaw.

A soft, sibilant sound will develop as the breath resonates, cutting away any nasal sound quality from now on. Listen to the breath, like the sound of gentle waves on the shore, and allow the breath to wash through the body, balancing every inhalation with an exhalation. It sounds a little like you are scuba-diving.

BANDHA TRAYAM – TRIPLE RESTRAINT

Bandha means lock or restraint and a bandha is a technique for locking or sealing energy into the body, which leads to improved health and vitality, physical strength and stamina, self-awareness and mental focus.

Core strength is developed, building internal support by working from deep inside the body. The body is protected and energized by the bandhas.

The muscles involved in harnessing these "locks" are both dynamic and subtle. Bandhas have far-reaching effects because they associate with the energy centres in the spine and the brain. Their contraction affects the nervous, circulatory, respiratory, endocrine and energy systems.

The development of bandhas in practising Astanga yoga is learnt over years, and in many yoga systems bandhas are not introduced until one is advanced in asana practice. To learn them you must work with a teacher.

JALANDHARA BANDHA

Restraining the jugular notch, by squeezing the glottis at the back of the throat, facilitates Ujjayi breathing. Narrowing the passageway like a valve, the breath is channelled, creating a sibilant, resonant sound, intensifying the cleansing effect of prana. The head is lifted and pulled back a little, thus stretching the neck and lengthening the spinal cord and the carotid sinuses are compressed.

BENEFITS:

This bandha helps to lower blood pressure and has great effects on the pituitary, pineal, thyroid and thymus glands in the endocrine system.

UDDIYANA BANDHA

Uddiyana bandha means flying upwards lock, referring to the lifting of the lower abdominal organs. The digestive organs are compressed by the action of hollowing the abdominal area from the pubic bone to the navel, creating an internal suction or vacuum.

To practise, keep the front ribs lifted, maintaining length in the front of your body. Concentrate on sealing the lower abdominal area towards the spine, hip bone to hip bone.

BENEFITS:

The subtle, sustained control of the lower abdominal muscles tones and revitalizes the digestive system and influences the adrenal glands and the pancreas, toning the kidneys and the solar plexus. The "brain in the stomach" is squeezed, forcing energy to shift and flood the abdomen and chest, which increases the gastric fire and cultivates lightness.

Uddiyana bandha brings vitality and youth, and is considered to be the most beneficial lock. It is described in the *Hatha Yoga Pradipika*, an ancient yogic text, as "the lion that conquers the elephant named death". On an esoteric level, it is said that Uddiyana bandha awakens kundalini energy which rises up the spine (see Chapter 8).

MULA BANDHA

Mula means root, source, or firmly fixed, and involves the conscious contraction of the perineum muscle, between the anus and the genitals. This "seat of power" activates the entire pelvic girdle of muscles, lengthening and protecting the lower back.

To practise, first contract all three muscles – urinary, genital and anus – in the pelvic floor and see if you can release them, isolating the middle muscle and keeping it gently lifted. This is the perineum and the root of the nervous system.

BENEFITS:

The support of this lift strengthens the reproductive glands and perineal body, bringing harmony to the genitourinary system. The nervous system is soothed, inducing calmness. It is said that, on an energetic level, Mula bandha connects with, and activates, the third-eye centre (see Chapter 8), so increasing concentration.

VINYASA – FOLLOW THE THREAD OF THE BREATH

Astanga Vinyasa yoga synchronizes the breathing system with deep stretching movements called vinyasas to let go of resistance in the body and mind.

The breath is the integrating link between mind and body, aligning them and facilitating a process of moving beyond physical and psychological barriers, which thus releases long-held stress and toxins.

Vinyasa means breath-connected movement. Like beads on a necklace, postures are threaded onto the breath in sustained meditative concentration. The flowing sequence detoxifies, stretches and lengthens muscles, and the heat created causes the blood to circulate and filter through the body's eliminative organs, shifting further toxins. As the above-mentioned alignment between mind, breath and body takes place, so dormant energy is liberated in a dance of tapas (intense discipline).

As one becomes absorbed in the flow of the practice, "new ways of thinking, new thoughts, come into your mind," says Pattabhi Jois.

DRISHTI – A SINGLE LINE OF FOCUS

An alert, steady gaze deepens concentration. There are nine gaze points, seven of which are in the primary series. They are named in the following practices, but do not strain to hold them. They are developed over time. First, learn the asana, alignment awareness and cultivate the bandhas and the breathing system.

The nine drishtis (gaze points) are: *Nasagrai* (nose), *Angusta ma dyai* (thumb), *Nabi chakra* (navel), *Padhayoragrai* (toes), *Hastagrai* (hand), *Parsva* (side), *Urdhva* (upwards), *Naitrayoh ma dyai* (centre eye, third eye), *Parsva Drishti* (far right or far left).

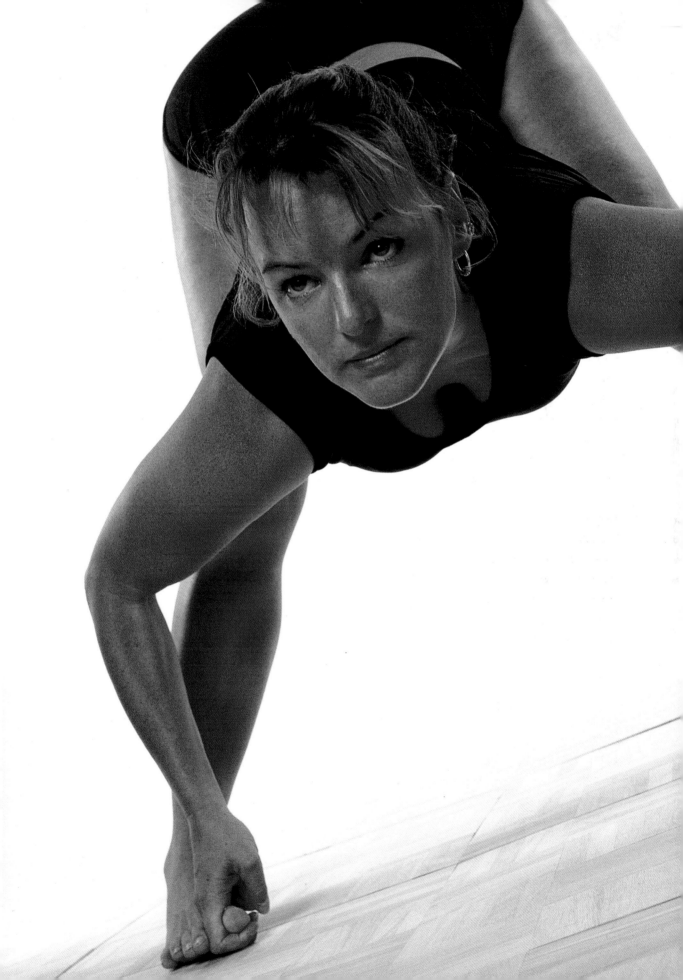

TAPAS (HEAT) – TRANSFORMING SPIRIT FROM MATTER.

Tapas, defined as "the concentration of the spiritual willforce", means to burn. It refers to the heat created from intense discipline, and is one of the Niyamas from the second limb of Patanjali's eight-limbed tree of yoga.

PHYSICAL TAPAS

Likened to heating up base metal to refine gold from ore, the body softens in the *Suryanamaskar* practice, becoming malleable and open, therefore unlocking safely. Burning off physical toxins in a process of physical tapas, perspiration strains off impurities through the largest organ of elimination, the skin.

MENTAL TAPAS

Focused attention on the breath, posture and gaze helps the mind to shift from the conscious to the subconscious realm, in a process of mental tapas. Through sustained concentration on the breath, psychic toxins are released, cultivating *swadhaya*, self-observation.

SPIRITUAL TAPAS

In a process of spiritual tapas, we begin to "pierce the veil" of *maya*, illusion, removing the "poison of conditioned existence" (as recited in the opening prayer – see page 1), by surrendering to a journey from ego to soul.

In other words, as we move from the gross (or manifest) world to the subtle (or unseen) world, we create the possibility of *Ishwara Pranadhanini*, which means "bowing to God".

ERASING SAMSKARAS

Our bodies can be a prison or a gateway to self-expression. Our past experiences are recorded in our bodies on a cellular level, and the emotions associated with them are called *samskaras*. Samskaras are imprinted in the voluntary nervous system like grooves on a record, and form our behavioural patterns, our tendencies – whether positive or negative – and, if unchecked, our addictions. They determine our life and colour our perception of the world, so we draw awareness to them and, little by little, we can release the patterns which are negative.

The vinyasa system involves stretching beyond the trammels of the mind, to transcend the conditioning of past habits. This process gradually lifts negative samskaras and erases them, giving us a clearer perception of the world and allowing us to change our belief systems.

Layer by layer, like peeling an onion, conditioning falls away.

The deepest aim of yoga meditation is to be able to rest, undistracted, in self-acceptance.

SURRENDER – SOFTEN THE MIND

The Tibetan expression for ego is *dak dzin*, and is translated as "grasping of the self". Pain is created when one resists the knowledge that only by learning non-attachment does one become free.

The practice of Astanga yoga is a metaphor for trusting the process of life and moving through fear and blockages, recognizing them as they arise and ending the struggle of holding on to them, i.e. the "grasping of the self".

Due to its dynamic nature, there can be a tendency to approach the practice of Astanga yoga competitively because of its challenging, exhilarating nature. It can become a narcissistic way of building yet more body armour rather than stripping away the muddy layers of ourselves to open the heart.

This is the antithesis of yoga, creating greater resistance in the mind and body, leading us away from ourselves, and the practice can become too "yang", or masculine, rather than seeking to balance the male and female aspects of ourselves.

We need to temper the practice with softness, in other words "yin", moon energy.

The ego controls; the soul surrenders. Trust the practice.

Pattabhi Jois repeats in class, "No fear... practise, practise, all is coming."

Let there be no scales to weigh your unknown treasure,

And seek not the depths of your knowledge with staff

or sounding line.

For Self is a sea boundless and measureless.

Say not, 'I have found the truth,'

But rather, 'I have met the soul walking along my path.'

For the soul walks along all paths.

The soul walks not upon a line, neither does it grow like a reed.

The soul unfolds itself, like a lotus of countless petals.

KAHLIL GIBRAN

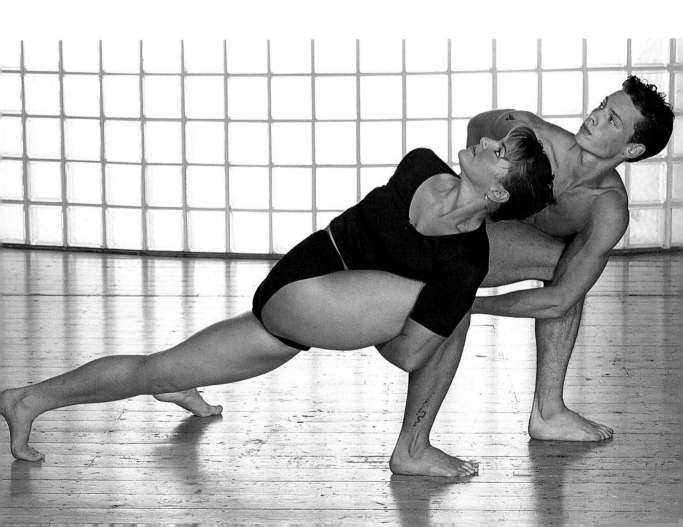

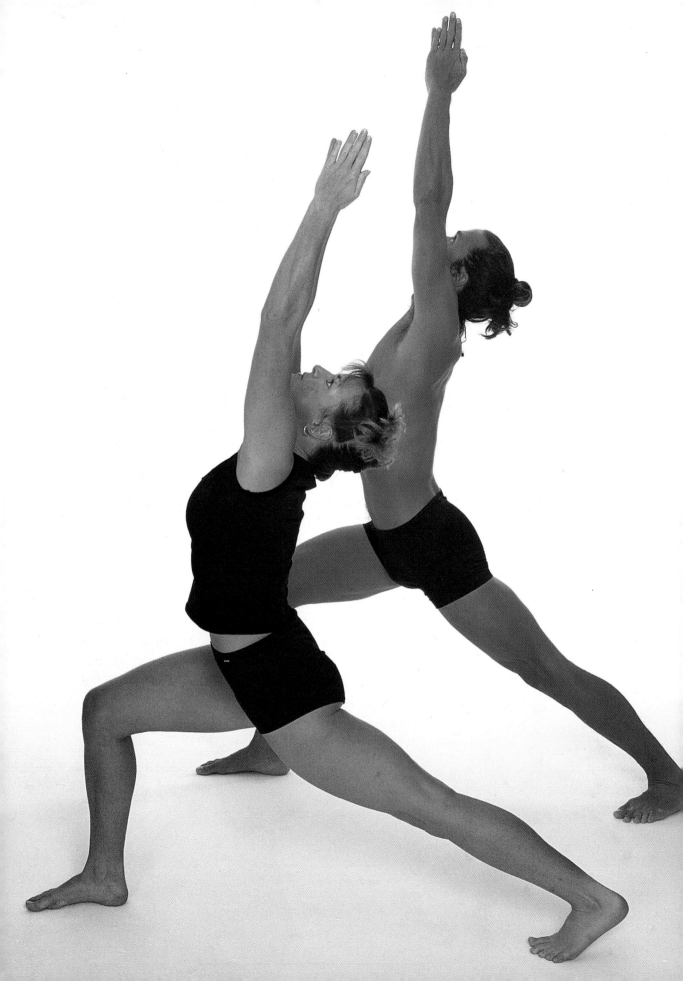

4

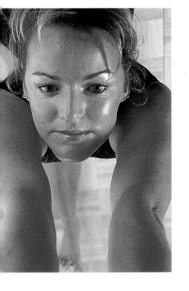

BEGINNING THE PRACTICE

This chapter presents the foundation postures and sequences which form the basis of the practice of Astanga Vinyasa yoga. We begin with the deeply energising exercise of Uddiyana bandha then continue with the two sun salutation sequences called Suryanamaskars. These are followed by the Standing Postures, a set sequence which realigns the body, increasing flexibility and building strength and stamina.

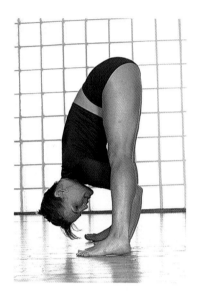

PREPARING FOR PRACTICE

Early morning or early evening are the ideal times to practise yoga. Morning is best, although the body may feel stiffer, but this is overcome with practice and through warming up.

It is preferable to practise on an empty stomach, otherwise leave approximately two hours after eating before you do any exercise.

As mentioned before, the yogic diet is *sattwic*, meaning that it should consist of fresh, vital, pure foods, which are as natural as possible. Traditional advice on eating is to fill half the stomach with food and a quarter with water, leaving a quarter for air, i.e. empty. And always aim to clear your bowels before you practise.

Try to remember the following points which will help you get the maximum benefit from your yoga session:

1. Always bathe before and after practising yoga.

2. Prepare the space you are using for your practice, and make sure it is clean and uncluttered. All you will need is yourself and a yoga mat.

3. Light a candle, or burn some incense or aromatherapy oil if you feel it will help you to focus.

4. Do not strain the body or the breath. Keep the brain soft and watchful.

CAUTION:

Do consult a doctor first, if you have, or have had, any of the following: cancer, MS, epilepsy, high blood pressure, recent surgery, a neck or knee injury, ear or eye problems, HIV or AIDS.

Blood pressure: all forward bends are soothing. B. K. S. Iyengar advises practising forward bends or the Downward Dog before and after inversions such as shoulderstands or headstands.

Eye/ear problems: avoid inversions.

Menstruation: rest for two days, this is a contemplative time, to encourage pratyahara, sense-withdrawal. A gentle practice of forward bends *(baddha konasana)* can ease heavy flow.

Pregnancy: practise with a specialist teacher. Rest for the first three months and don't apply any pressure on the abdomen. *Baddha konasana* and *upavistha konasana* are excellent to free tightness in the pelvis and lower back.

Knees: be careful not to overextend your knees. Always make sure the direction of the knee follows the direction of the foot and work on encouraging flexibility in the hips, not on forcing or straining the knees.

OPTIONS FOR PRACTICE

The hardest part of the practice is beginning it! But it is said that the journey of a thousand miles begins with a single step...

If you have 20 minutes: practise five rounds of Suryanamaskara A and B, followed by the finishing sequence and relaxation (see Chapter Six).

If you have 45 minutes: practise from the beginning, do five rounds of Suryanamaskara A and B, the standing postures, and the finishing sequence (see Chapter Six) followed by a period of relaxation.

If you have 90 minutes: you should do the full Primary Series (Chapters Four, Five and Six). Practise from the beginning, doing five rounds of Suryanamaskara A and B, and the standing postures, then add the Primary Series postures, one by one, following the method, and end with the Finishing Sequence, then relax. If you cannot complete the full Primary Series, close the practice at Navasana, the Boat posture, then go to the Finishing Sequence. If you cannot get into a full asana, just work to the edge of your ability, stopping at stages 1 or 2 as outlined, and BREATHE there, releasing into the asana as the body unlocks. Let emotions surface. Notice precautions and modifications where appropriate.

Do not attempt the advanced postures without guidance from a teacher.

The stages listed below guide us systematically through the Astanga Vinyasa yoga practice. The next part of this chapter covers stages 1-4. Stages 5-7 are dealt with in Chapters Five, Six and Seven respectively.

1. Uddiyana bandha (flying-up lock)

2. Suryanamaskara A (First Sun Salutation)

3. Suryanamaskara B (Second Sun Salutation)

4. Standing Postures: Foundation of the Practice

5. Primary Series: Seated Postures

6. Finishing Postures: Backbends/Inverted postures.

7. Relaxation

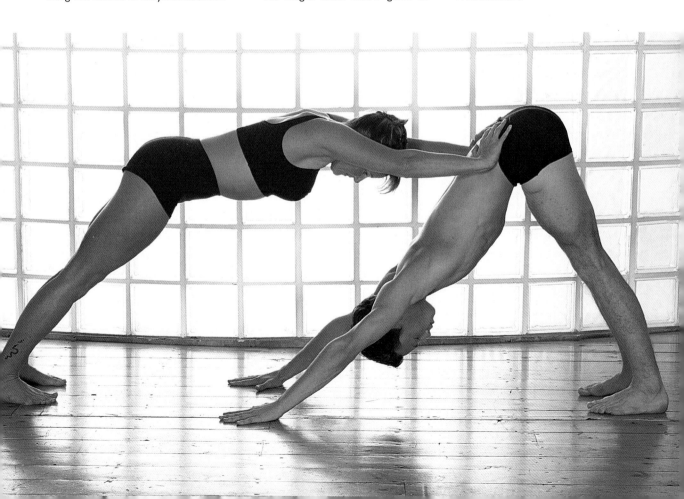

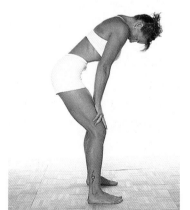

UDDIYANA BANDHA – PRELIMINARY PRACTICE

1. Stand with your feet apart, bend your knees and lean slightly forwards. Press your palms on to the middle of your thighs, spreading your fingers, keeping your spine and arms straight.

2. Inhale deeply, and then push the exhalation out of your lungs, emptying them. Allow your body to lean forwards as you do this (1).

3. Retain the exhalation, do not inhale!

4. Draw your abdominal wall inwards towards your spine, sucking your navel in, to create a hollow beneath the floating ribs. With straight arms and spine, press your palms into the thighs (2).

5. Maintain this position for a few seconds. Then release the hold, inhaling deeply, and follow with some resting breaths.

6. Repeat five times.

CAUTION:

Do not repeat this exercise more than once a day.

Only practise it on an empty stomach. Do not practise it if you have an IUD, are pregnant, or menstruating.

BENEFITS:

This powerful, energizing exercise nourishes the abdominal organs, shifting sluggish energy and toxins, and stimulates digestion. It is not part of the primary series, but is an optional preliminary practice.

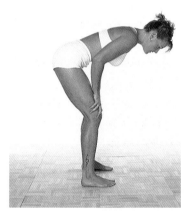

TADASANA (MOUNTAIN POSE) – THE FIRST CLASSICAL ASANA

1. Stand at the front of the mat, placing your feet together (the inner sides of the ankles and big-toe joints should be just touching). Spread the balls of your feet wide, open your toes like a fan, and ground all four corners of your feet.

2. Seal your muscles on to the bones of your legs, by lifting your kneecaps and thigh muscles upwards. Check that your kneecaps are facing directly forwards.

3. Lift your upper body out of the pelvis, centring your body either side of the spine. Tuck your tailbone down and lengthen (or stretch) your spine upwards, keeping your neck long, through to the base of your skull. Lengthen your abdomen, feeling your ribcage floating above your pelvis.

4. Breathe deeply into your side-ribs.

5. Widen your collarbones, broad-ening across the top of your chest and soften your shoulders away from your ears, but keep your armpits lifted.

6. Press down through the soles of your feet and, keeping your neck long, lift the crown of your head towards the sky. Feel a polarity stretch within your body, i.e. from your pelvis down, root into the earth, and from your pelvis upwards, lift your upper body towards the sky.

7. Look straight ahead of you with a soft gaze, as if looking towards an imaginary horizon.

BENEFITS:

The art of good posture and body awareness begins here. The posture cultivates awareness of alignment and balance, supporting the spine and skeletal structure of the body, and allowing the internal organs to sit correctly.

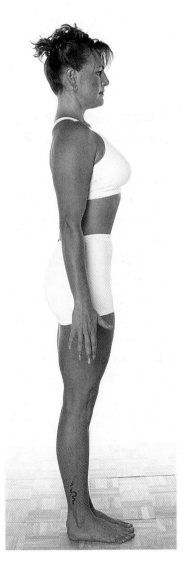

BREATH AND BANDHAS

UJJAYI BREATHING

Begin to lengthen each breath, as explained in Chapter 3 (see page 29), consciously balancing each inhalation and exhalation. Expand each inhalation into your side-ribs, keeping your shoulders relaxed. This throat lock is called Jalandhara bandha.

UDDIYANA BANDHA

Drop your mind into your abdomen, and on the next exhalation, gently draw the wall of the abdomen towards your spine from the pubic bone upwards, hollowing the lower belly. From hip bone to hip bone, seal in the lower abdomen, cultivating Uddiyana bandha.

MULA BANDHA

Begin to lift the muscles in your pelvic floor, more specifically, the perineum muscle, to support the floor of your torso. This is Mula bandha, the root lock (see page 30 for more detail).

From now on, our aim is to sustain these three inner grips – Jalandhara bandha (the throat lock), Uddiyana bandha (the abdominal lock) and Mula bandha (the root lock) – and channel the Ujjayi breath throughout the practice.

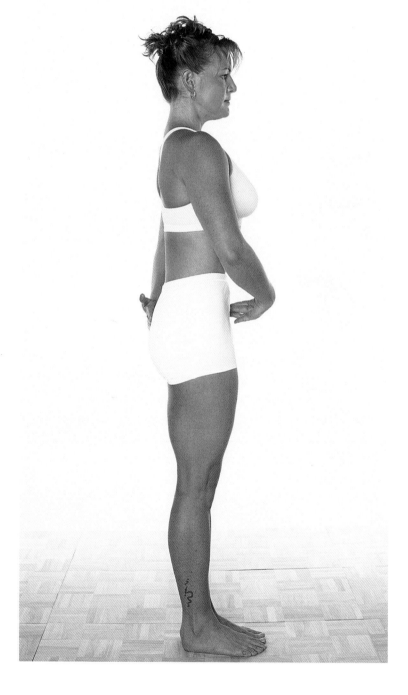

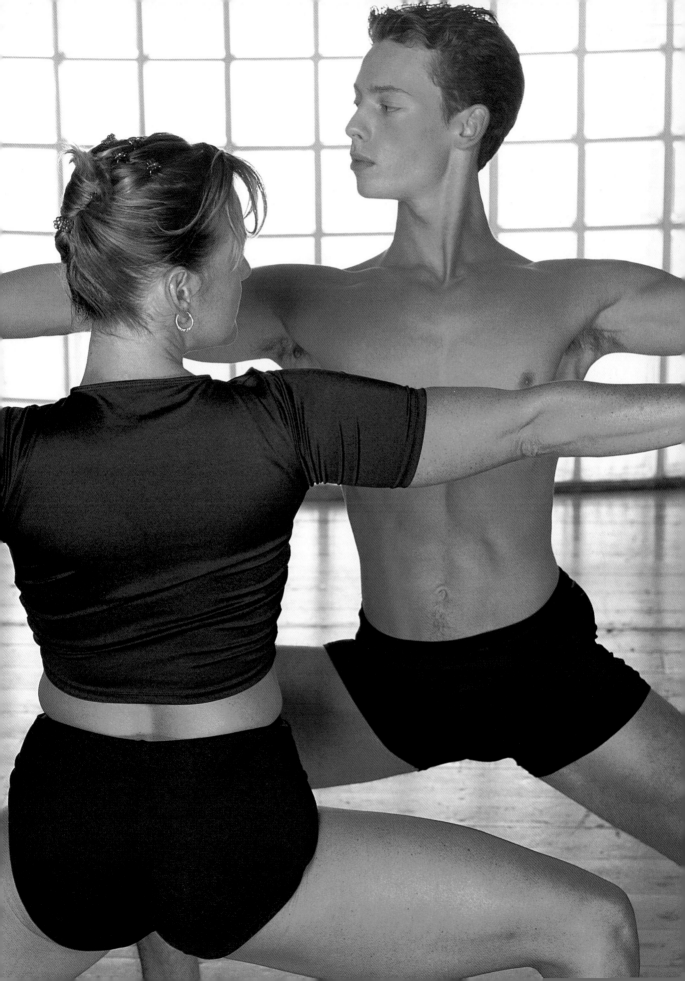

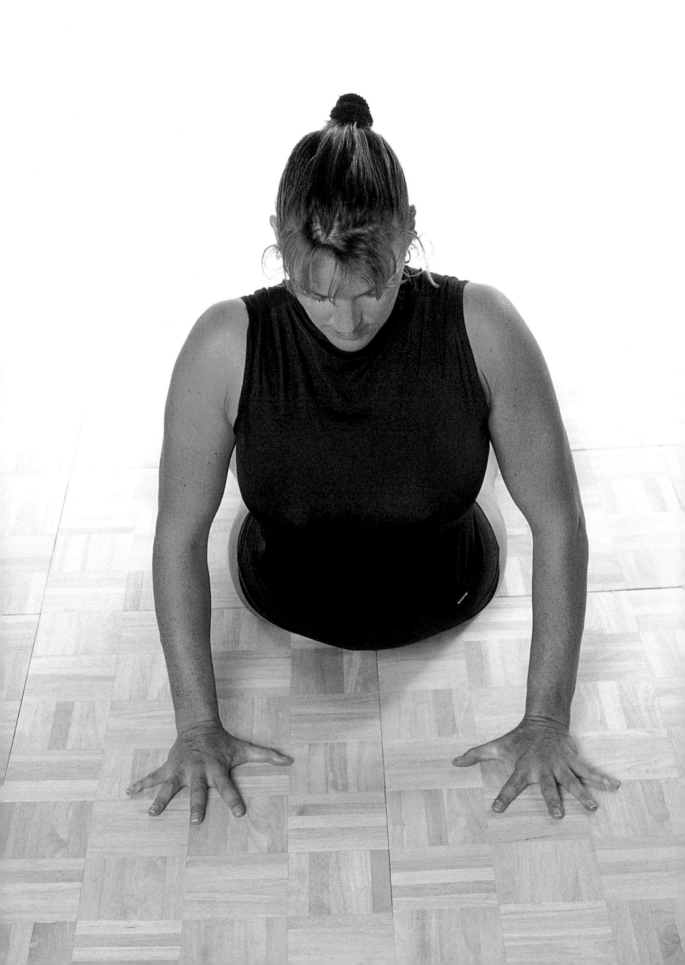

Suryanamaskara A – Salute to the Sun – is the opening sequence in Astanga yoga, threading postures on to the breath, warming up the body for practice, cultivating concentration, a deep focus, positive intention and alignment. The sun salutations build heat and sweat to detoxify the body and prepare it to stretch safely into deep postures.

There are two Suryanamaskar sequences: the first (A) consists of ten movements, which stretch and awaken the spine. The second, Suryanamaskara B, is a development on the first, adding two new postures – Utkatasana (the Fierce posture) and Virabhadrasana (the Warrior pose) – which work deeper into the hips, deepening alignment and concentration. Together they stretch and tone the body in artful sculpting.

SURYANAMASKARA Ⓐ

While learning the following sequence, take five breaths in each posture, in order to attain a feeling of a deep stretch and alignment awareness. Do not rush. Keep breathing. Once you have learnt each posture, build up a continuous sequence on the thread of each breath, sustaining only the Downward Dog for five breaths. (If necessary, rest in the Cat or Child's posture.)

The following pictures illustrate how the sequence flows through each posture and the vinyasas which link the postures together. The pictures are then repeated with instructions on how to move into each posture. Always begin in the first classical posture of Tadasana.

Repeat the sequence five times until you can maintain the flow of breathing, so creating vinyasa, or breath-synchronized movement, as well as building tapas (heat) and cultivating concentration.,

BENEFITS:
Suryanamaskara concentrates the mind, making the body strong and flexible, shedding tension and stiffness.

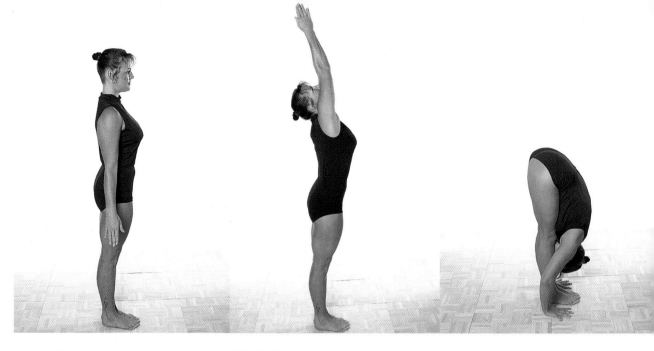

Tadasana CENTRE YOUR BODY AND CONNECT TO THE CORE.

ekam 1 INHALE, RAISE YOUR ARMS AND LOOK UP TO YOUR THUMBS.

due 2 EXHALE, LOWER YOUR BODY AND GAZE TOWARDS THE TIP OF YOUR NOSE, THEN MOVE INTO UTTANASANA.

SURYANAM

panca 5 INHALE, ROLL YOUR BODY OVER YOUR TOES, MOVE INTO THE UPWARD DOG POSTURE AND LOOK UP.

sat 6 EXHALE, ROLL YOUR WEIGHT OVER YOUR TOES, MOVE INTO THE DOWNARD DOG, LOOK TOWARDS YOUR NAVEL AND TAKE FIVE BREATHS.

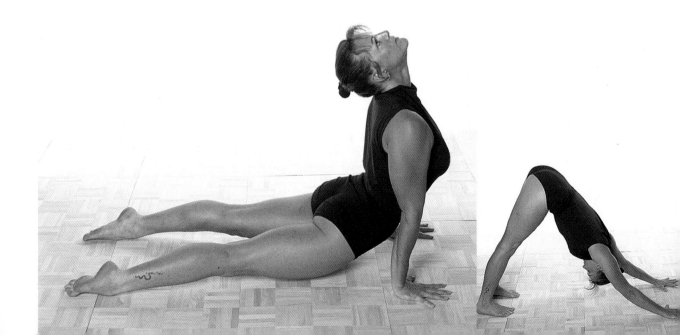

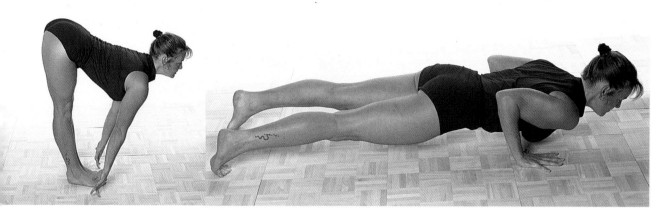

trini 3 INHALE, LIFT YOUR CHEST AND LOOK UPWARDS. THIS IS URDHVA UTTANASANA.

catvari 4 EXHALE, JUMP BACK, LOWER YOUR CHIN TOWARDS THE FLOOR AND MOVE INTO CHATURANGA DANDASANA (THE STAFF POSE).

A S K A R A

sapta 7 INHALE, BEND YOUR KNEES AND LOOK UP.

astau 8 JUMP YOUR FEET SO THAT THEY END UP BETWEEN YOUR HANDS, EXHALE, BEND FORWARDS AND MOVE INTO THE UTTANASANA POSITION.

nava 9 INHALE, RAISE YOUR ARMS UP AND LOOK UP. EXHALE, AND RETURN TO TADASANA.

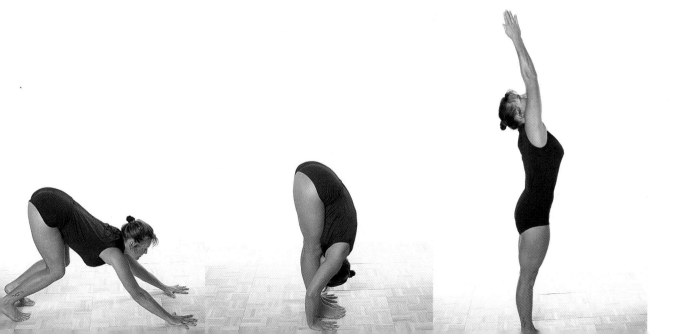

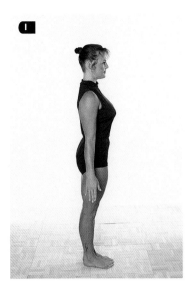

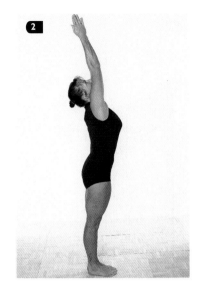

Tadasana (Mountain): Centre your body, connecting to your core. Keep your tailbone tucked down and your lower belly hollowed to protect the lower back.

Raised Tadasana: Inhale, raise your arms up sideways over your head. Press the palms together and look up to your thumbs. Breathe. Your arms should reach up like an arrow.

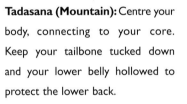

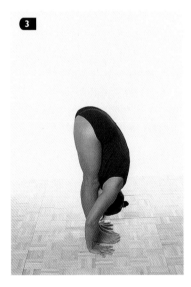

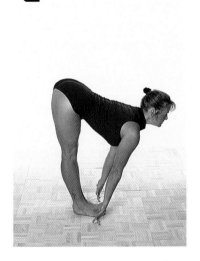

Uttanasana (intense stretch): Exhale, fold your body forwards, lengthening and releasing your spine. If possible, allow your abdomen to touch your thighs. Drop your head to lengthen your neck.

Urdhva Uttanasana: Inhale, look up, lift your chest and lengthen the wall of your abdomen.

Place your hands beside your feet, with palms pressed down, fingers spread wide like a starfish (not shown).

5

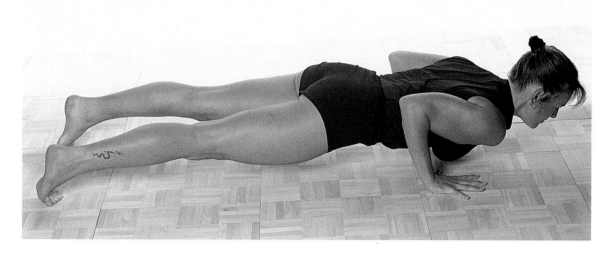

Chaturanga Dandasana (Four-angled Staff or Staff pose): Exhale, step or jump your feet back into Diagonal Plank, by placing your feet hip-width apart. Keep your back straight and strong in line with your legs. Your arms should be fully extended and your lower abdomen drawn inwards, creating a diagonal line through your body. Inhale, keep your abdomen drawn back, your legs strong. Exhale, then gently lower your body to the floor, bending your elbows and pressing them into your side-ribs, while keeping your legs strong and straight. Your hands should be pressed, palms downwards, close beside your ribcage. (If this is too intense, lower your knees first, then your body. Do not strain your back.) Tuck your toes under and press your palms deep into the mat beside your side-ribs. Making your body strong and straight, lift first your legs off the floor, then your abdomen, third your chest, creating a straight line. This may take some time. Just practise! (If it is too hard, keep your chest touching the floor when necessary.) Keep breathing!

6

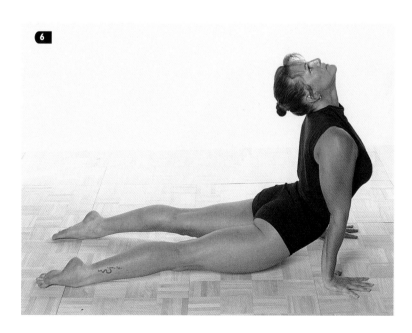

Urdhva Mukha Svanasana (Upward Dog): Inhale. If your toes are tucked under, roll over them, arching your spine. Then look up, with only your hands and the tops of your feet touching the floor. Work your legs, squeezing the muscles on to the bones, and straighten your arms and open your chest.

(If this is too intense, keep your legs touching the floor, but strengthen them and arch your spine, keeping your elbows bent a little. Do not strain your back – strong legs should support the back.)

7

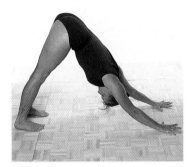

8

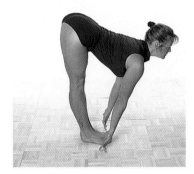

Ardho Mukha Svanasana (Downward Dog): Exhale, roll over your toes, pushing your hips up to the sky and pressing your heels towards the floor. Lengthen your spine, lift your front ribs away from your pelvis, hollowing your lower belly. Push away from your hands and straighten your legs. Press the palms of your hands down, especially the inside edges and stretch your fingers open like a starfish. Drop your chin to your chest to release your neck. Take five deep Ujjayi breaths.

Uttanasana: Inhale, bend your knees and look up. Jump, or step your feet together between your hands, and exhale. Fold your head into your knees, releasing your spine. (If you have pain in your back, soften and bend your knees.)

mod

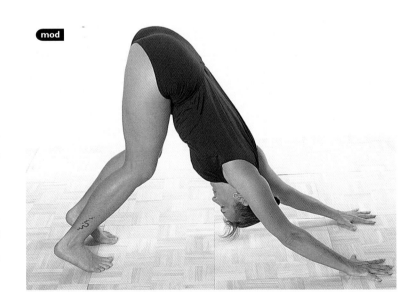

If this is too intense, bend your knees, drawing your belly on to your thighs **(mod)**.

If your wrists are strained, or you have back pain, drop your knees to the floor and repeat ten rounds of the Cat posture, then lift your hips to return to the Downward Dog pose.

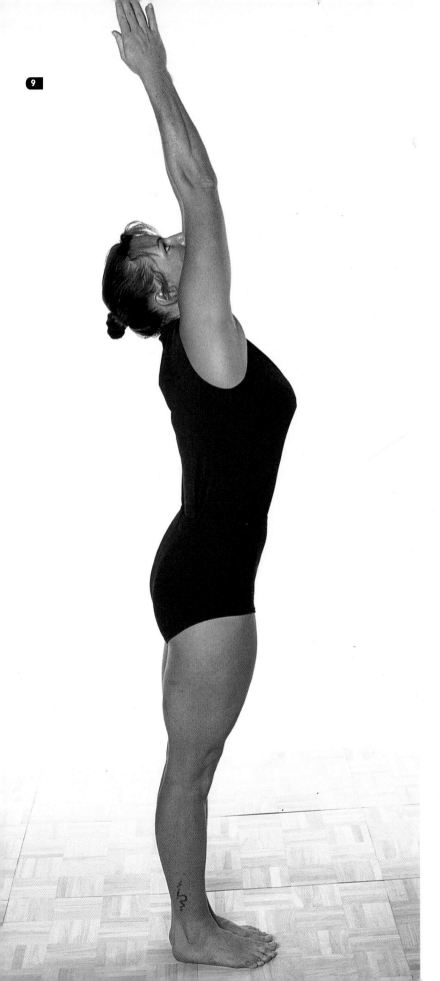

9

Raised Tadasana: Inhale, raise your arms in a sideways movement up over your head, press the palms of your hands together and look up.

10

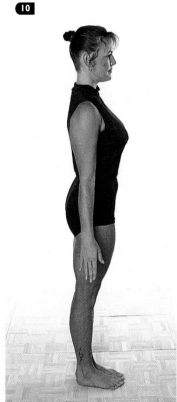

Tadasana: Exhale and return the arms to the sides to Mountain pose.

Repeat Suryanamaskara A five times, following the thread of the breath, linking it with the movements.

DRISHTIS (GAZE POINTS) FOR SURYANAMASKARA A: THUMB, NOSE AND NAVEL

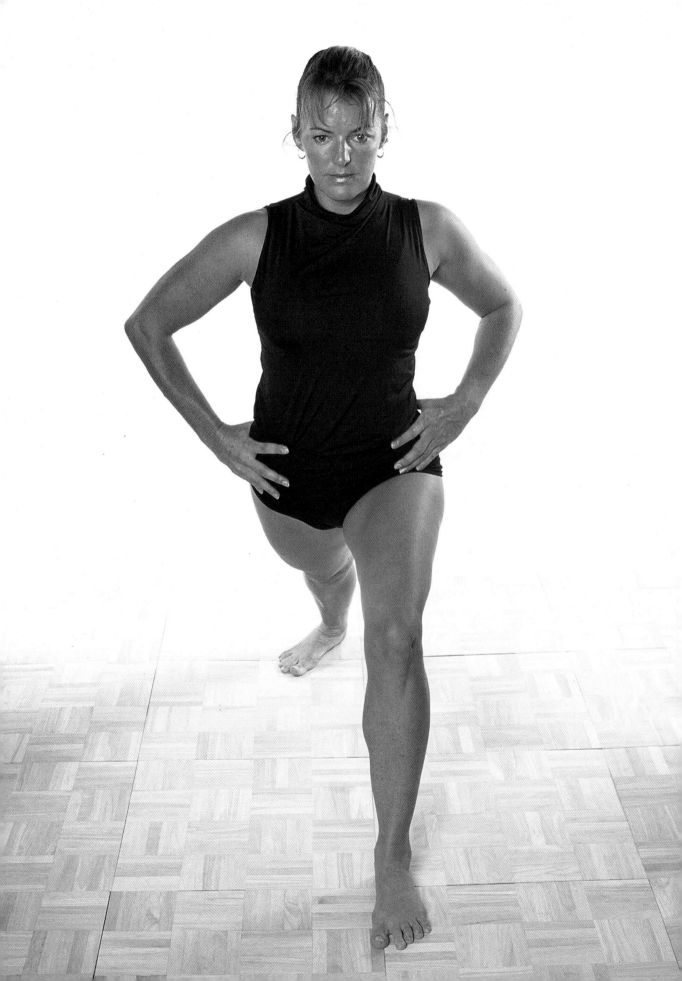

SURYANAMASKARA Ⓑ

In the second sun salutation, we add two new postures: Utkatasana (the Fierce pose) and Virabhadrasana A (the Warrior posture). The pictures on the next four pages demonstrate how Suryanamaskara B moves through a flowing sequence based on Suryanamaskara A. The sequence is developed, but having mastered Suryanamaskara A, much of it will be familiar. Once you have looked at the flow of the movements, you can practise them by following the instructions for each in more detail.

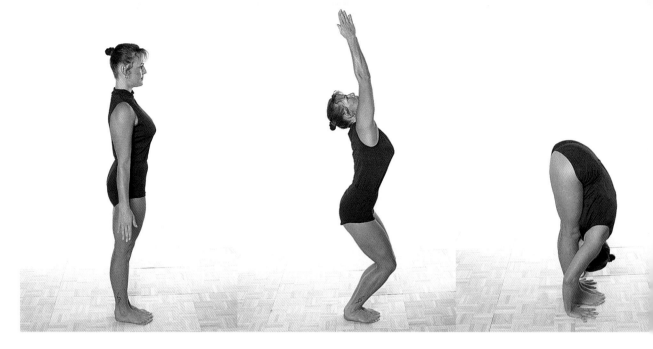

Tadasana BEGIN IN TADASANA. FOCUS AND, BREATHING DEEPLY, DRAW YOUR LOWER ABDOMEN TO YOUR SPINE AND LIFT THE ROOT LOCK.

ekam 1 INHALE. MOVE INTO UTKATASANA, THE FIERCE POSE. DROP YOUR HIPS, RAISE YOUR ARMS AND LOOK UP.

due 2 EXHALE, FOLD YOUR UPPER BODY FORWARDS AND GAZE TOWARDS THE TIP OF YOUR NOSE, MOVING INTO UTTANASANA.

SURYANAM

panca 5 INHALE, ROLL YOUR BODY OVER YOUR TOES, MOVE INTO THE UPWARD DOG POSE AND LOOK UP.

sat 6 EXHALE, ROLL YOUR BODY OVER YOUR TOES AGAIN AND MOVE INTO THE DOWNWARD DOG POSE.

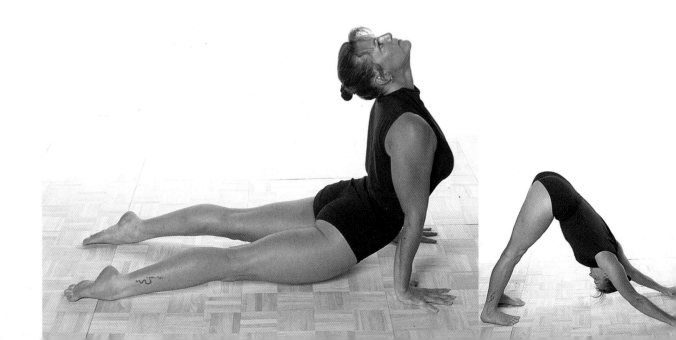

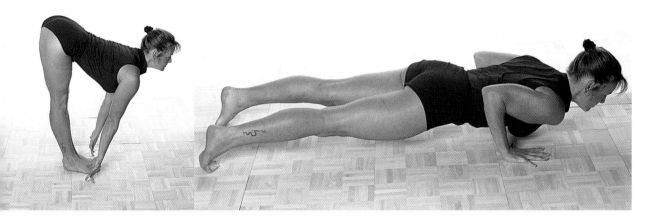

trini 3 INHALE, LIFT THE CHEST UP AND LOOK UP, MOVING INTO URDHVA UTTANASANA.

catvari 4 EXHALE, JUMP BACK, LOWER YOUR CHIN TOWARDS THE FLOOR AND MOVE INTO CHATURANGA DANDASANA.

A S K A R A Ⓑ

sapta 7 INHALE, MOVE INTO VIRABHADR-ASANA A, PIVOTING THE LEFT HEEL IN AND TAKING THE RIGHT FOOT FOR-WARDS . RAISE YOUR ARMS UP AND LOOK UP.

astau 8 EXHALE, MOVE INTO CHATURANGA DANDASANA.

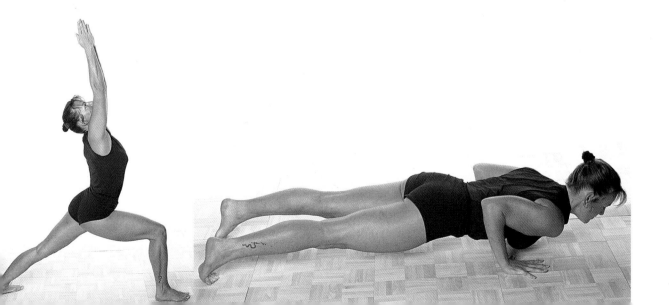

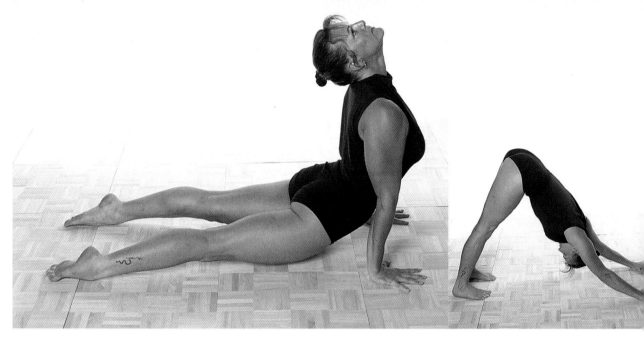

nava 9 INHALE, ROLL OVER YOUR TOES, LOOK UPWARDS AND MOVE INTO UPWARD DOG POSE AND LOOK UP.

dasa 10 EXHALE, ROLL BACK OVER YOUR TOES AND MOVE INTO DOWNWARD DOG. LOOK TOWARDS YOUR NAVEL.

S U R Y A N A M

traydasa 13 INHALE, ROLL OVER YOUR TOES, LOOK UPWARDS, MOVE INTO UPWARD DOG AND LOOK UP.

caturdasa 14 EXHALE, ROLL OVER YOUR TOES, LOOK DOWN TOWARDS YOUR NAVEL AND MOVE INTO DOWNWARD DOG. TAKE FIVE BREATHS.

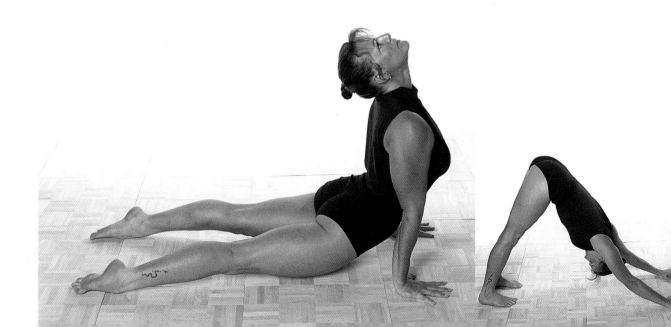

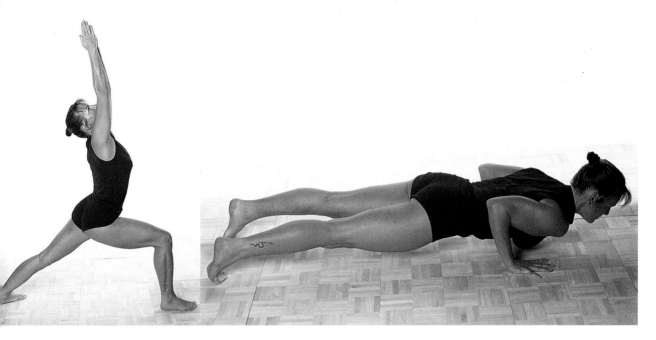

ekadasa 11 INHALE, AND MOVE INTO VIRABHADRASANA A. THIS TIME PLACE YOUR LEFT FOOT FORWARDS BETWEEN YOUR HANDS. RAISE YOUR ARMS AND LOOK UP.

dvadasa 12 EXHALE, MOVE INTO CHATURANGA DANDASANA, LOWERING YOUR CHIN TO THE FLOOR.

A S K A R A Ⓑ

pancadasa 15 INHALE, BEND YOUR KNEES AND LOOK UP (KEEP YOUR HIPS RAISED HIGH).

sodasa 16 EXHALE, JUMP YOUR FEET BETWEEN YOUR HANDS, FOLD FORWARDS, MOVING INTO UTTANASANA AND EVENTUALLY DROP YOUR HEAD.

saptadasa 17 INHALE, MOVE INTO UTKATASANA, DROPPING YOUR HIPS DOWN, RAISING YOUR ARMS AND LOOKING UP. EXHALE AND RETURN TO TADASANA.

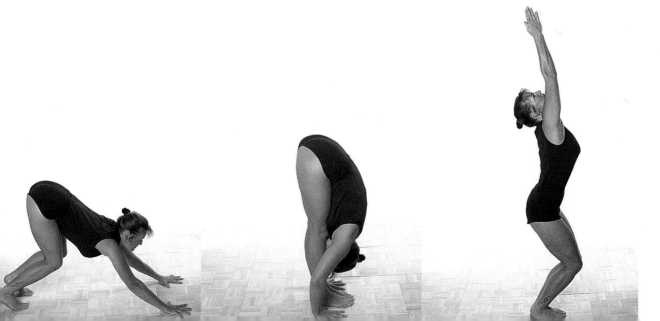

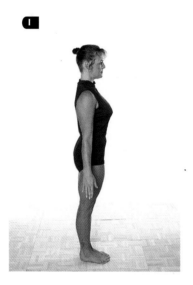

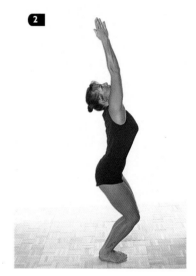

Tadasana: Stand in Tadasana. Lengthen your spine upwards, breathing deeply.

Ground your feet, press the inner seams of your legs together and lift the crown of your head. Draw your navel to your spine and lift the root lock **(1)**.

Utkatasana (Fierce pose): Inhale, reach your arms up over your head, and drop your pelvis as if sitting into a chair. Gaze towards your thumbs,

and hollow your lower belly **(2)**.

Uttanasana (Intense pose): Exhale, and fold your body forwards out of your hips, keeping your knees soft as you release your spine over your thighs. Inhale, lift your chest and look up (see page 46).

Chaturanga Dandasana (Staff pose): Exhale, lightly jump (or step) back into Staff pose. (If this is too intense, lie on the mat.)

Urdhva Mukha Svanasana (Upward Dog): Inhale, roll over your toes into Upward Dog and arch your spine.

Ardho Mukha Svanasana (Downward Dog): Exhale and roll over your toes into Downward Dog, pushing your hips back and pressing your heels to the floor. Take one full breath.

Virabhadrasana A (Warrior Pose): (Virabhadrasana means

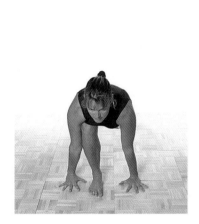

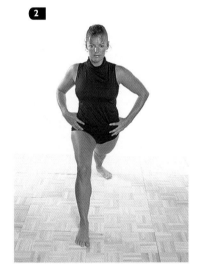

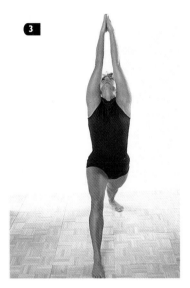

Powerful Hero posture.) Inhale, turn your left heel into your right big toe. Exhale and place your right foot between your hands **(1)**.

Lift your upper body and bend into your right thigh, bringing your body parallel to the floor.

Place your hands on your hips and, using your hands like a steering wheel, draw your right hip back and encourage your left hip forwards **(2)**.

Keep breathing as you "set", i.e.

align, your body. Draw your stomach inwards between your front hip bones, and open out your . chest. Keep breathing. Share your weight equally between both legs as if you are sitting in a saddle. Lift the root lock. Inhale, raise your arms over your head, press the palms of your hands together and look up **(3)**.

Breathe deeply. This is Virabhadrasana, the Warrior pose. Lift your upper body out of your pelvis and lengthen the arms like an arrow.

Chaturanga Dandasana: Exhale, lower your arms beside your front foot and jump (or step) back into Staff pose. Empty your lungs.

Upward Dog: Inhale, roll over your toes into Upward Dog, arching your spine.

Downward Dog: Exhale, roll over your toes into Downward Dog, pushing your hips back and pressing your heels to the floor. Take one full breath.

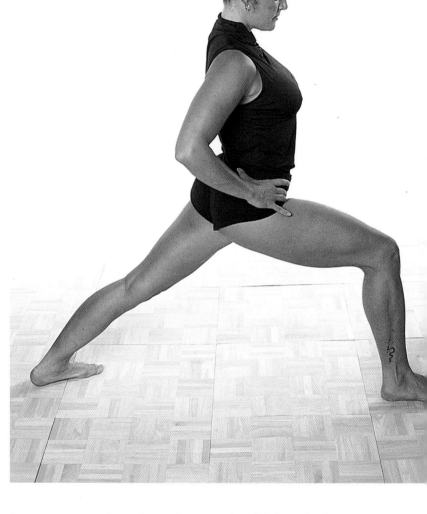

Virabhadrasana A (Second Side): Inhale, turn your right heel into your left big toe. Exhale, and place your left foot between your hands. Lift your upper body, bending deeply into your left thigh, bringing it parallel to the floor. Place your hands on your hips, encouraging the right hip to rotate forwards and the left hip to drop back. Inhale deeply into the bottom corners of your lungs and raise your arms over your head. Pressing your palms together, look up.

Chaturanga Dandasana: Exhale, lower your arms beside your front foot, stepping back into Staff pose. Empty your lungs.

Upward Dog: Inhale, roll over your toes into Upward Dog (rest your chest on the floor if necessary while you are learning), arching your spine.

Downward Dog: Exhale, roll over your toes, press your hips back and lift your pubic bone. Press your heels down to open your hamstrings and calf muscles and take five deep breaths.

Uttanasana: Inhale, bend your knees, and look up. Then exhale, jump or step your feet between your hands and fold into Uttanasana, the deep forward bend.

Utkatasana: Inhale, bend your knees, raise your arms over your head, gaze at your thumbs and press your palms together. Exhale and release your arms, returning to Tadasana.

Repeat Suryanamaskara B five times, aiming to achieve an unbroken flow choreographed to the Ujjayi breathing. If you are a beginner, repeat the sequence slowly, taking as many breaths as you need in order to find depth in each posture. Aim to build a sense of fluidity in your movements.

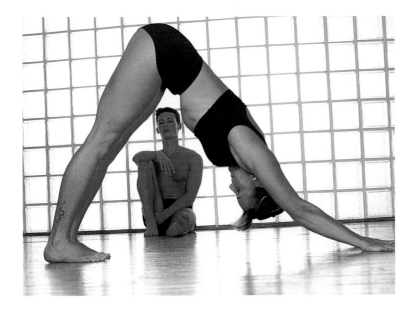

Downward Dog: This also resembles a dog stretching, but in this asana the whole of the back (west side) of the body is nourished, thus releasing the shoulders and neck. It is excellent for hamstrings, calves and the Achilles tendons. It strengthens the ankles and shapes the legs, while healthy blood flows to the torso and brain, slowing the heart.

Virabhadrasana A: This shapes, strengthens and tones the legs and back. It also massages the abdominal organs. Helping to realign the hips, this posture releases stiffness in the shoulders, back, ankles, knees and hips. It opens the chest, encouraging deep breathing, and helps to slim hips and cultivate stability.

DRISHTIS FOR SURYANAMASKARA B: THUMB, NOSE, NAVEL.

BENEFITS:

Uttanasana: This asana tones the liver, kidneys and stomach and can help alleviate period pain. It is also a good tonic for the heart and spine, and soothes the brain.

Utkatasana: This unlocks the shoulders and develops the chest. It strengthens and aligns the legs, ankles and thighs, as well as toning the back, heart and abdominal organs.

Chaturanga Dandasana: This tones the abdominal organs, and helps to strengthen the upper body and wrists.

Upward Dog: Resembling a dog stretching, the whole of the front (east side) of the body is stretched, rejuvenating the spine, expanding the chest and opening the lungs. Healthy blood flows to the pelvic region.

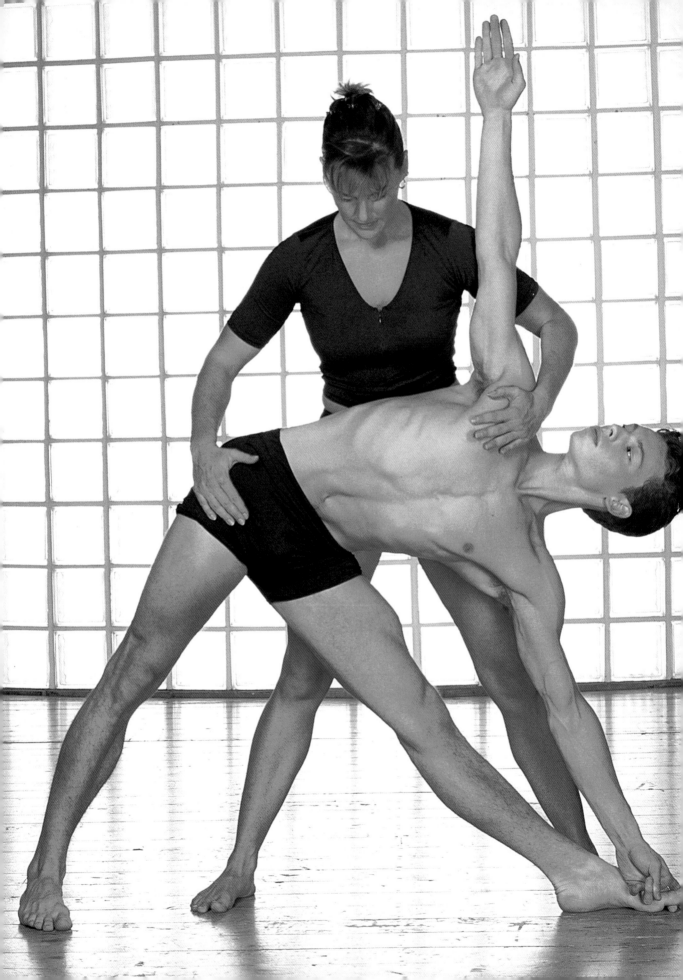

STANDING POSTURES

The Standing Postures develop strength, flexibility and stamina. They powerfully realign the spine, balancing the left and right sides of the body, bringing flexibility to the hips, spine and shoulders. The sequence, however advanced one is, always follows the same form and you will see why as you experience the benefits. As in all Hatha yoga practice, the asanas conform to a pattern of stretches. The first are forwards, the second backwards, and the third lateral (sideways), while the fourth are twists, the fifth balances and the sixth inversions (which appear towards the end of the practice). These key directions all contribute to stretching the body and awakening the spine.

PADANGUSTHASANA (FOOT-TOE) – CATCHING THE TOES

DRISHTI (GAZE POINT: NOSE

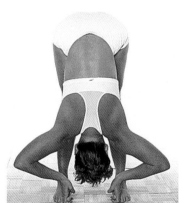

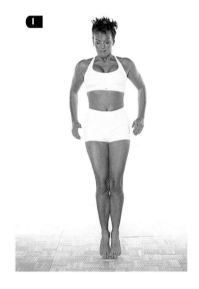

1. Inhale, jump your feet hip-width apart **(1)**, Place your hands on your hips. Exhale, spread your toes and square the outsides of your feet.

2. Inhale, lift your chest and look up **(2)**.

3. Exhale, fold your upper body from the front pelvis into a forward bend, catching the toes. The first two fingers should hook round the neck of the big toes **(3)**.

4. Inhale, pull on your toes and look up, lengthening your abdomen and sealing it inwards **(4)**.

5. Exhale, fold your body right over the thighs and release your spine into a forward bend. Take five Ujjayi breaths.

6. Breathe deeply and do not force your upper back or shoulders. Aim to touch your thighs with your abdomen. If necessary, keep your knees bent. Don't force your body or your breathing, but release your spine with every exhalation.

7. Inhale, lift your chest and look up.

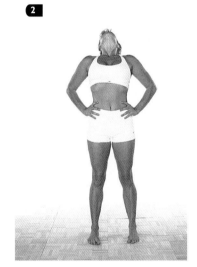

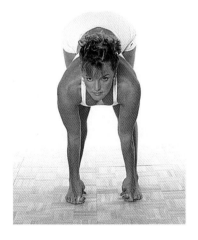

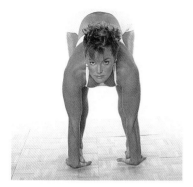

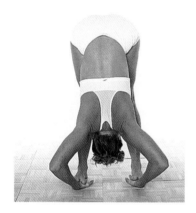

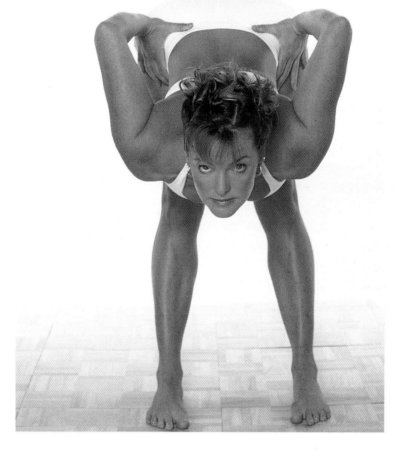

PADDAHASTASANA – STAND ON THE HANDS

DRISHTI: NOSE

Padda means foot and *hasta* means hands.

1. Exhale and stand on your hands with your toes facing the inner part of your wrists.

2. Bend your knees to achieve the release of the lower back, if necessary. Inhale, lift your chest and look up (**1**).

3. Exhale, fold the body deeper, drawing your chin between your knees (**2**).

4. Breathe mindfully, balancing every inhalation with the corresponding exhalation.

5. Point your sitting bones up and lengthen your spine with every exhalation. Take five Ujjayi breaths.

6. Inhale, lift your chest and look up. Then exhale and place your hands on your hips. Draw your abdomen towards your spine and open your shoulders. Inhale, come up and look up (**3**).

7. Exhale, jump back into Tadasana (Mountain pose), pressing your feet together. Centre your body and take one full breath.

BENEFITS:

These postures help tone the abdomen and spine, resting the internal organs and heart. They have a calming effect which helps to combat depression.

UTTHITA TRIKONOSANA – EXTENDED TRIANGLE

DRISHTI: HAND

1. Inhale, jump to the right, so your feet land parallel, 3ft apart. Exhale, lift your chest and roll back your shoulders **(1)**.

2. Inhale, turn your left toes inwards 15 degrees, keeping your left outside heel grounded

3. Exhale, rotate the ball of your right foot outwards 90 degrees. Draw back your left hip and ground your left foot. Inhale and lengthen your spine **(2)**.

4. Exhale and tilt your body to the right, keeping your left hip and left shoulder drawn back.

5. Keep breathing and hook your right big toe with your right hand **(3)**. If this is not possible, hold your right leg instead. Look up to your left thumb, and open the palm of your hand **(4)**. Keep your neck long, drawing your chin to your left shoulder. Take five Ujjayi breaths.

Now repeat the posture on the left side.

1. Inhale and return to the starting position. Then exhale and rotate your right foot inwards 15 degrees and your left foot out 90 degrees.

2. Draw back your right hip and shoulder. Inhale, lengthen your spine, and open your chest.

3. Exhale, tilt your upper body to the left, catching your left leg or big toe of your left foot. Keep your right hip drawn back and widen the space between your front hip bones.

4. Reach your right arm up and turn your gaze to your top thumb. Breathe freely, and roll back your right shoulder. Take five Ujjayi breaths.

BENEFITS:

This stretch tones the waist and hips. Strength and flexibility are developed in the legs, ankles and hips, while it also shapes the legs and develops the chest. It relieves backaches and neckaches.

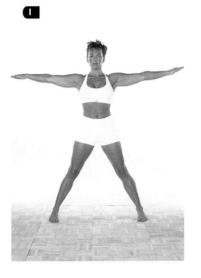

1

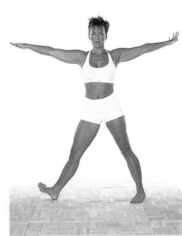

2

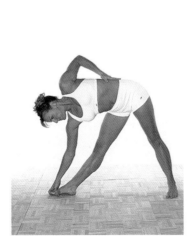

3

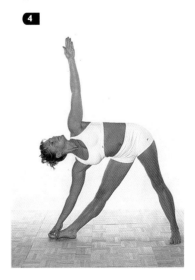

4

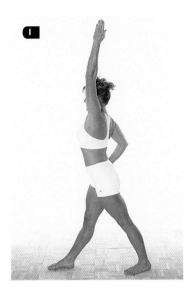

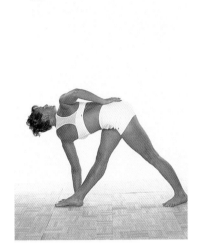

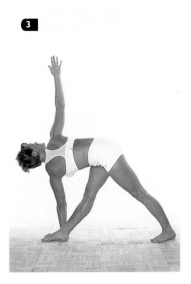

PARIVRTTA TRIKONASANA – REVOLVED TRIANGLE

DRISHTI: HAND

1. Inhale, press into the outer edge of your right foot as you come up.

2. Exhale, place your hands on your hips and pivot your pelvis to the right. Facing over your right thigh, use your hands like a steering wheel and push your right hip back.

3. Inhale, lift your left arm up, stretching your left waist **(1)**. Then exhale and extend your upper body out of your pelvis, placing your left hand outside your right foot. If it doesn't reach, place your hand on your right leg.

4. Inhale, place your right hand on your sacrum and twist your spine, drawing back your right shoulder and your right hip **(2)**.

5. Exhale and extend your right arm

to the sky **(3)**. Look up to your thumb. Breathe deeply, lift your lower abdomen towards your spine, and seal your muscles on to the bones of your legs, keeping them strong and straight. Take five Ujjayi breaths.

Now repeat the posture on the left side:

1. Inhale and return to the centre position.

2. Exhale and rotate your pelvis to face over your left thigh. Keep your right foot grounded and your legs firm.

3. Inhale and raise your right arm up, stretching the right side of your waist. Exhale, extend your upper body out of your hips and place your right hand outside your left foot (or on your leg).

4. Inhale, draw back your left hip, roll open your left shoulder, and place your left hand on your sacrum.

5. Exhale and reach your left arm up towards the sky, with your palm open, and gaze towards your thumb. Take five Ujjayi breaths.

6. Inhale, press into the edge of your right foot and come up. Exhale, bend your knees and lightly jump back into Tadasana. Take one full breath.

BENEFITS:

Twisting, nourishing and strengthening the spine, this posture also massages the internal organs and aids the elimination of waste matter. Ankles, knees, thighs are toned, the chest is developed, and the waist and hips slimmed.

UTTHITA PARSVAKONASANA - EXTENDED SIDE-ANGLE

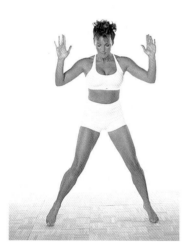

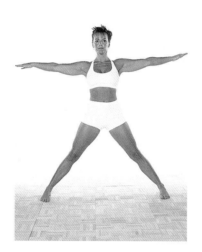

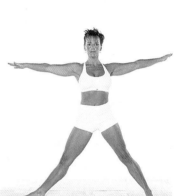

DRISHTI: HAND

1. Inhale, jump to the right, gently landing with your feet about 4ft apart **(1 & 2)**. Ground your feet and spread your toes. Exhale, roll back your shoulders and open your chest lengthening your spine.

2. Inhale, turn your left foot in 15 degrees, then exhale and turn your right foot out 90 degrees **(3)**.

3. Inhale, draw back your left hip and ground your left foot. Exhale and bend your right leg deeply until your thigh is parallel to the floor. Root into your left foot, sharing equal weight between both legs. Inhale, lengthen your spine and open your chest.

4. Exhale, keeping your left shoulder drawn back, place your right hand outside your right foot **(4)**. Press your right knee into your armpit, creating a straight line between your right shinbone and your right arm. Inhale and raise your left arm over your head.

5. Exhale and extend your arm over your head, creating a diagonal stretch through the left side of your body **(5)**. Breathe into your side-ribs and press the edge of your back foot down. Draw back your left shoulder and your left hip. Take five Ujjayi breaths.

Now repeat the posture on the left side:

1. Inhale and come back to the centre position. Exhale, lengthen your

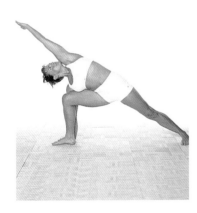

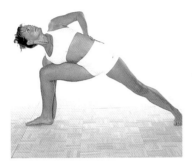

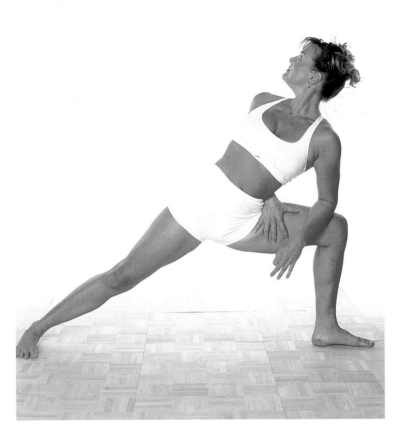

spine and harness the bandhas.

2. Inhale and rotate your right foot in 15 degrees. Exhale, turning your left foot out 90 degrees. Inhale and draw back your right hip, grounding your right foot.

3. Exhale, bend your left leg to a 90-degree angle and place your left hand outside your left foot. Press your knee into your armpit and create a straight line between your shinbone and arm.

4. Inhale and raise your right arm over your head.

5. Exhale and extend your arm over your head to create a diagonal stretch through the right side of your body. Breathe into your side-ribs and ground your right foot. Then take five Ujjayi breaths, gazing at the middle finger.

MODIFICATION:

Right Side: Keeping your left shoulder open, sit your right elbow on your right thigh **(mod)**. Draw your left hand behind you to catch your inner right thigh. Turn your chin to your left shoulder, broadening your chest. Open the left side of your body as deeply as you can.

Reverse these instructions for the left side.

BENEFITS:

This posture gives a deep lateral stretch which shapes the waist and legs, tones the thighs, ankles and knees and develops the chest. It also aids the elimination of waste matter.

PARIVRTTA PARSVAKONASANA – REVOLVING SIDE-ANGLE

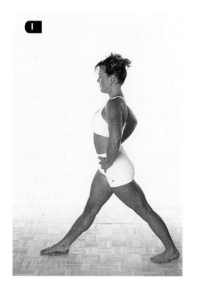

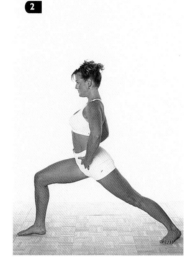

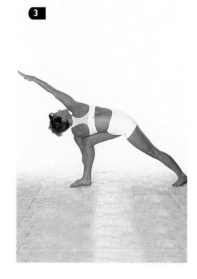

DRISHTI: HAND

1. Inhale and come up to the original starting pose, with your feet about 4ft apart. Place your hands on your hips.
2. Exhale and pivot your pelvis to face right. As you turn, rotate the ball of your left foot inwards 15 degrees, and turn your right foot out 90 degrees **(1)**. Inhale, open your chest and stretch out your front body,
3. Exhale and bend your right leg to a right angle **(2)**. Inhale and draw your left arm outside your right thigh, to create a lever for the pose.
4. Place your hands in the namaste prayer position (i.e. over your heart) with your right elbow pointing up. Drop your right hip back, aiming to get your thigh parallel to the floor. Press your left foot into the mat. Take five Ujjayi breaths.
5. If possible, place your left hand outside your right foot, draw your right shoulder back, and stretch your right arm up and over your head **(3)**.

Now repeat the posture on the left side:

1. Inhale, come up into the centre and place your hands on your hips.
2. Exhale and pivot your pelvis to the left. Rotate the ball of your right foot in 15 degrees and turn your left foot out 90 degrees. Inhale and lengthen your front body.
3. Exhale and bend your left leg to a deep right angle. Then inhale and lift your right arm **(4)**.

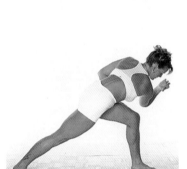

4

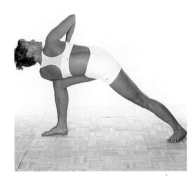

mod

BENEFITS:

This is an addition to the Primary Series which I include because it gives such a fantastic twist. It works deeper in terms of internally massaging organs. The colon is massaged, the liver detoxified and digestion stimulated. Blood flows to the spine, nourishing the back muscles, and the waist, ankles, knees and thighs are toned.

CAUTION:

If you have vulnerable knees, bend them a little as you practise to check you are not locking them. Support your joints by lifting your kneecaps and thighs, sucking your muscles on to the bones of your legs. Check that your kneecap always follows the direction of your foot. Keep a sense of fluidity in your joints by imagining space in them.

4. Exhale and place your right shoulder outside your left thigh and your right hand outside your left foot. Inhale, open your chest and look up.
5. Exhale and stretch your left arm up and over your head and gaze towards your middle finger. Take five Ujjayi breaths, channelling the breath through the throat lock.

MODIFICATION:

The full posture takes some practice. Stay with the modification, concentrating on making your legs strong and firm, and rotating your hips until you are able to manage the deep twist, with your shoulder outside your opposite thigh.

Right side: Place your hands into the namaste prayer position with your right elbow pointing up **(mod)**. Draw your right hip back, so that your right thigh is parallel to the floor.

Reverse the instructions for the left side.

At the end of each posture inhale, come up, exhale and return to Tadasana.

A1

A2

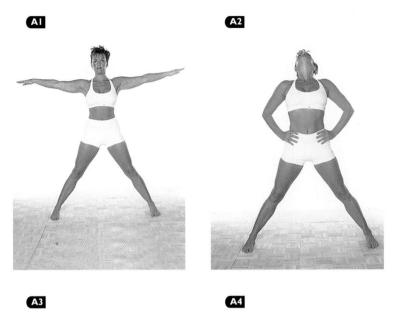

A3

A4

PRASARITA PADOTTANASANA - EXPANDED LEG INTENSE STRETCH

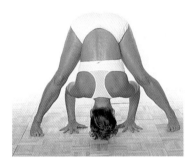

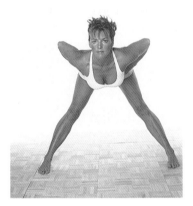

DRISHTI: NOSE

There are four variations of this posture, which I have labelled A to D.

A

1. From Tadasana, bend your knees and, as you inhale, jump to the right with your feet parallel. Do not turn them outwards. Spread the balls of your feet wide and splay the toes. Ground your big-toe joints, the little toe edges, the inner and outer heels

and charge your legs, drawing the muscles onto the bones. Lengthen your spine and open your chest. Inhale and extend your arms out wide **(A1)**.

2. Exhale and place your hands on your hips; then inhale, lift your chest and look up **(A2)**.

3. Exhale and fold your body from your front pelvis, touching the floor with your hands. Place your hands in line with your feet and make sure your legs are wide enough to press

your palms into the mat **(A3)**.

4. Inhale, look up and straighten your spine. On the next exhalation, release into a forward bend again, breathing fully, and lift your front ribs away from your pelvis. Take five Ujjayi breaths in this position.

5. Inhale and look up; then exhale and place your hands on your hips, drawing your abdomen back towards your spine **(A4)**. Inhale and come up; then exhale and release your hands to your sides.

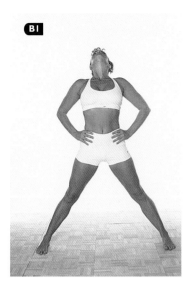

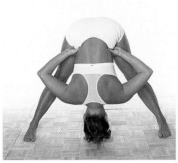

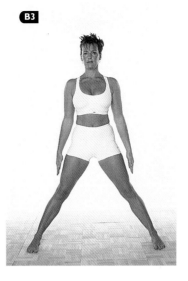

B

1. Start in the same position as for A.

2. Inhale and extend your arms wide.

3. Exhale and place your hands on your hips .

4. Inhale, lift your chest and look up (**B1**).

5. Exhale, fold your body forwards from your front pelvis, keeping hands on hips, and bring your head to the floor (**B2**).

6. Take five deep Ujjayii breaths.

7. Inhale and come all the way up.

8. Exhale and release your arms to your sides (**B3**).

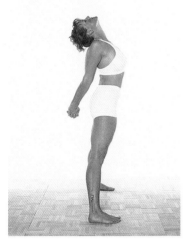

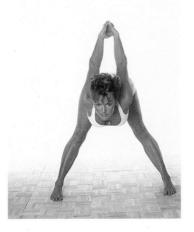

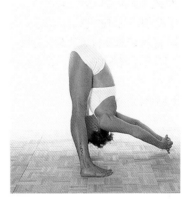

C

1. Start in the same position as for version A.

2. Inhale and extend your arms wide.

3. Exhale and clasp your hands behind your back, interlocking your fingers. Inhale, lift your chest and look up (**C1**).

4. Exhale and fold your body forwards from your front pelvis (**C2**), drawing your arms up over your head towards the floor behind you.

Your palms should be facing into your body. Take five breaths, think your head down to the floor (**C3**).

5. Inhale and come all the way up.

6. Exhale and release your arms to your sides.

D1

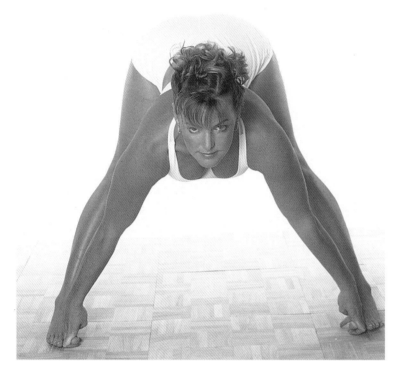

D2

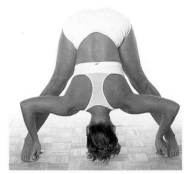

D

1. Start in the same position as for version A.

2. Inhale and extend your arms wide.

3. Exhale and place your hands on your hips.

4. Inhale, lift your chest and look up.

5. Exhale and fold your body forwards from your front pelvis. Hook each big-toe joint with the first two fingers of each hand, with your palms facing in.

6. Inhale and pull on your toes, lift your chest and look up **(D1)**.

7. Exhale and draw your body forwards, aiming to keep your abdomen long and your spine as straight as possible. Do not bow your thorax or tighten your shoulders. Take five breaths, and with every exhalation release your spine, widening the space between each vertebra **(D2)**.

8. Inhale and look up; then exhale and place your hands on your hips.

9. Inhale and come all the way up; and, finally exhale, release your arms to your sides and jump your feet back to Tadasana. Focus your gaze, or drishti, straight ahead of you, ground your feet, and stretch up through the core of your body.

BENEFITS:

This sequence of standing postures strengthens the legs and opens hamstrings. Blood flows to the upper body and head, nourishing the brain. All the standing poses help to balance and reduce body weight.

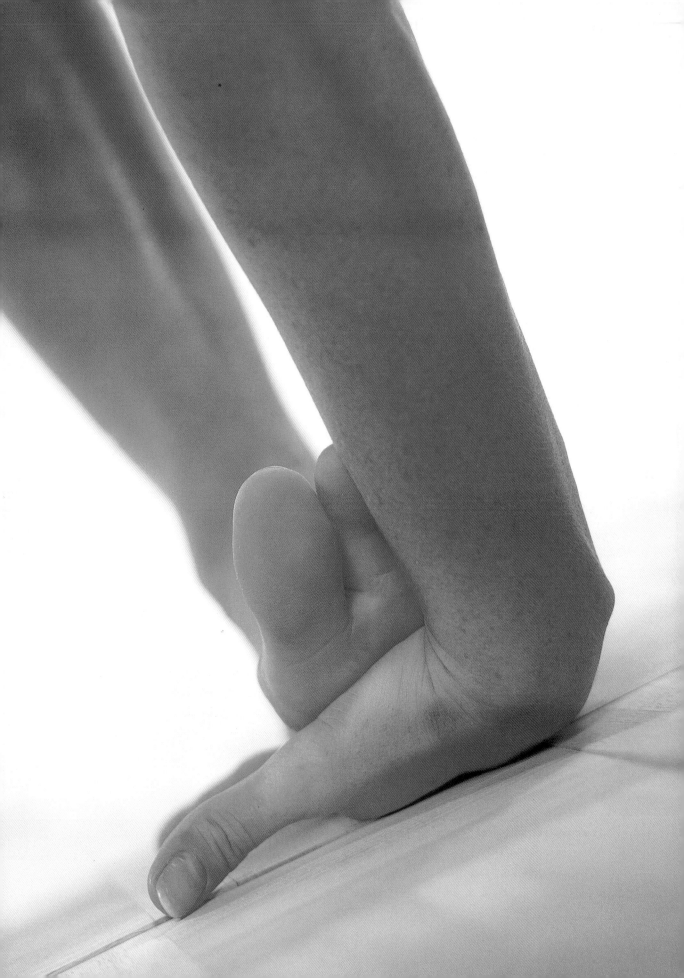

PARSVOTTANASANA – INTENSE SIDE STRETCH

DRISHTI: NOSE

1. From Tadasana, inhale, bend your knees and jump to the right.

2. Exhale as you land with your feet 3ft apart and your arms wide. Inhale and bring your arms behind you. Exhale and press your palms together in the reverse namaste prayer position, fingers pointing up and with the edges of your hands pressed into your spine. Keep your chest open and your shoulders drawn back.

3. Inhale and pivot the ball of your left foot inwards 15 degrees; then exhale and pivot the ball of your right foot outwards 90 degrees. Draw back your right hip, turning your pelvis to face over your right thigh. Keep your legs strong and your muscles drawn up (1).

4. Inhale and lean back, lengthening the front of your body and opening your shoulders and chest (2).

5. Exhale and extend forwards out of your hips, making a deep fold over your right thigh. Keep your spine long, lengthening your abdomen and drawing your navel to your spine (3). Drawing your chin to your shin, gaze at your big toe and ground your big - toe joint. Aim to align your spine over your extended leg. Draw back your shoulders and lift your chest. Take five Ujjayi breaths, channelling your breath through Jalandhara bandha (4).

Now repeat the posture on the left side:

1. From the posture you are already in, inhale and come up. Exhale.

2. Follow the instructions for this stretch as in the initial steps 3, 4 and 5, this time pivoting the ball of your right foot inwards 15 degrees and the ball of your left foot outwards 90 degrees.

3. At the end, exhale, release your arms and jump lightly back to the Mountain posture.

BENEFITS:

This posture opens the hips, shoulders and wrists. The legs are made strong and supple, and the spine is awakened.

MODIFICATION:

If your arms are too strained, fold your elbows behind your back instead.

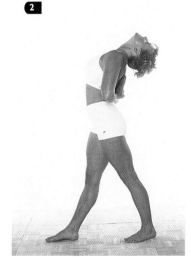

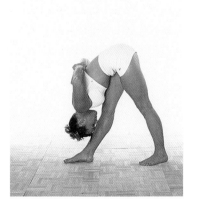

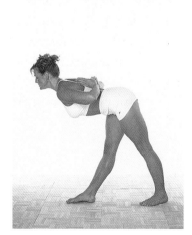

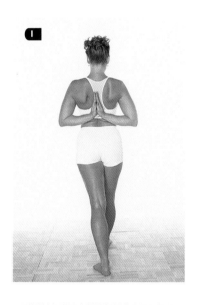

UTTHITA HASTA PADANGUSTHASANA – EXTENDED HAND, FOOT AND BIG TOE

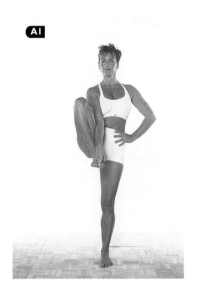

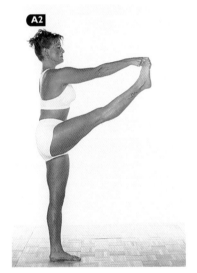

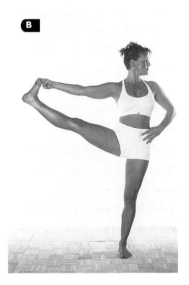

DRISHTI: TOES AND FAR RIGHT AND FAR LEFT.

There are four stages of this posture which I have labelled A, B, C and D for ease. Instructions for the right side are given first.

A

1. From Tadasana, root into your left foot, spreading your toes and charging your left leg. Place your left hand on your left hip. Inhale and raise your right leg to catch either your shin or your big toe **(A1)**. Aim to straighten both legs **(A2)**. The same principles of alignment apply – stretch up out of your pelvis, open your top chest, and broaden out your collarbones. Seal your navel to your spine and lift your pelvic floor. Take five Ujjayi breaths.

B

1. Exhale, and with your raised right leg either bent or straight, open your hip, drawing your leg to the right, and turn your gaze to the left **(B)**. Keep your spine long and stay strong in your back, drawing open your left shoulder.
2. Take five Ujjayi breaths.

C

1. Inhale, bring your right leg back to the centre and hold on to your foot, ankle or heel with both hands.
2. Then exhale, centre your body and square your hips
3. Inhale and raise your right leg as high as you can. Keep your hips parallel **(C)**.

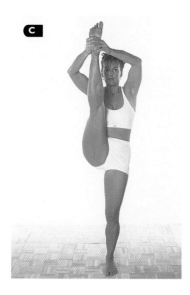

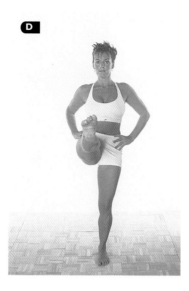

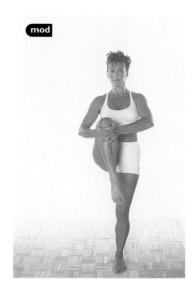

D

1. Exhale and place your hands on your hips, and keep your right leg raised, pointing your toes **(D)**. Use abdominal strength to support your back and your raised right leg. Sustain for five deep breaths, finding energy in your breath and bandhas.

5. Exhale, release the position and realign in the Mountain pose.

Now repeat the posture on the left side:

A

1. From Tadasana, root into your right foot, spreading your toes and charging your right leg and place your right hand on your right hip.

2. Inhale and raise your left leg to catch either your shin or your big toe. Take five Ujjayi breaths.

B

1. Exhale and with your raised left leg bent or straight, draw your leg to the left, and turn your gaze to the right. Keep your spine long and your chest open, drawing open your right shoulder. Take five Ujjayi breaths.

C

1. Inhale, bring your raised left leg back to the centre and hold on to your ankle or heel with both hands.

2. Exhale, centre your body and square your hips.

3. Inhale and raise your left leg as high as you can, keeping your hips level. Take five Ujjayi breaths.

D

1. Exhale and place your hands on your hips, and keep your left leg raised, pointing your toes. Use abdominal strength to support your back and your left leg. Find energy in your breath and bandhas. Take five Ujjayi breaths.

5. Exhale, release and realign yourself in the Mountain pose.

BENEFITS:

This posture shapes the legs and cultivates steadiness, balance and poise.

MODIFICATION:

Practise the posture with your knee bent, hugging your shin **(mod)**. Just take one breath in stages 3 and 4 of the leg raise. The alignment is the most important thing, not how high you raise your leg. Keep your back straight and balance the left and right sides of your body.

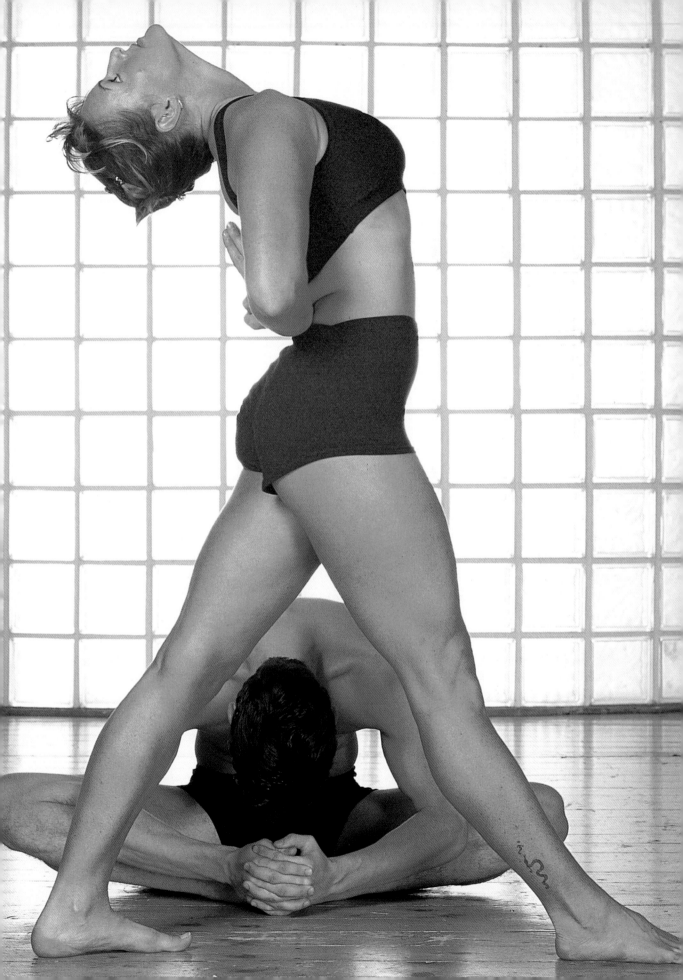

1

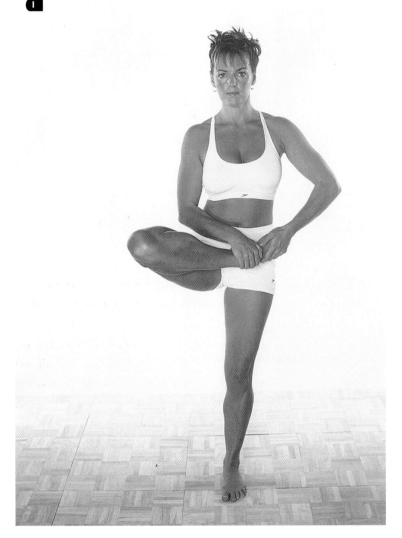

2

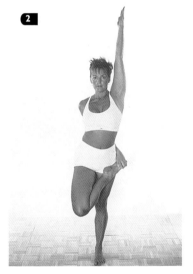

ARDHA BADDHA PADMOTTANASANA – HALF-BOUND LOTUS INTENSE FORWARD BEND

DRISHTI: NOSE

If you are attempting this posture for the first time, practise the version given under Modification (see opposite).

1. Ground your left foot and raise your right leg, sealing your shinbone on to your thigh bone. Rotate your right hip as you drop your knee towards the floor, and bring your right heel high towards your navel.

2. Inhale and place your right foot into a half Lotus **(1)**. Do not force your knee (see Modification opposite). If you are an advanced yoga practitioner, bind the Lotus by bringing your right hand behind your back and catching the big toe of your right foot.

3. Inhale and stretch your left arm upwards, keeping the crown of your head towards the sky **(2)**.

4. Exhale and come forward, placing your left hand on the floor outside your left foot with your palm flat on the ground **(3)**. Take five Ujjayi breaths.

5. Inhale and look up; then exhale and bend (soften) the standing knee.

6. Inhale and come all the way up;

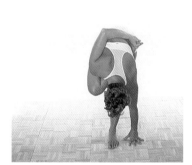

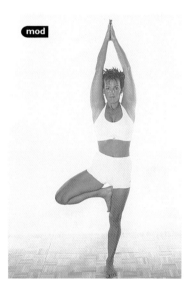

the ground. Take five Ujjayi breaths.

5. Inhale and look up; then exhale and bend (soften) the standing knee.

6. Inhale and come all the way up, and finally exhale, release your leg and return to the Mountain posture.

MODIFICATIONS:

Press your right foot to your left inner thigh, as high as possible. Charge the standing leg, squeezing your muscles on to your bone.

Draw your right knee as far back as possible and lengthen your spine. Place your hands into the namaste prayer position at chest level, then raise your arms like an arrow **(mod)**.

Please do not strain your knees!

BENEFITS:

Practising this posture tones and stengthens the legs, bringing balance and poise. The meditative quality of the balancing poses cultivates the "third eye", i.e. intuition or inner vision.

then exhale, release your leg and return to the Mountain pose.

Now repeat the posture on the left side:

1. Ground your right foot and raise your left leg, sealing your shinbone on to your thigh bone. Rotate in your right hip joint as you drop your knee towards the floor, and bring your left heel high towards your navel.

2. Inhale and place your left foot into a half Lotus. Do not force your knee.

If you are an advanced yoga practitioner, bind the Lotus by bringing your left hand behind your back to grasp the big toe of your left foot.

3. Inhale and stretch your right arm upwards, drawing the crown of your head towards the sky.

4. Exhale and fold forward, placing your right hand on the floor outside your right foot with your palm flat on

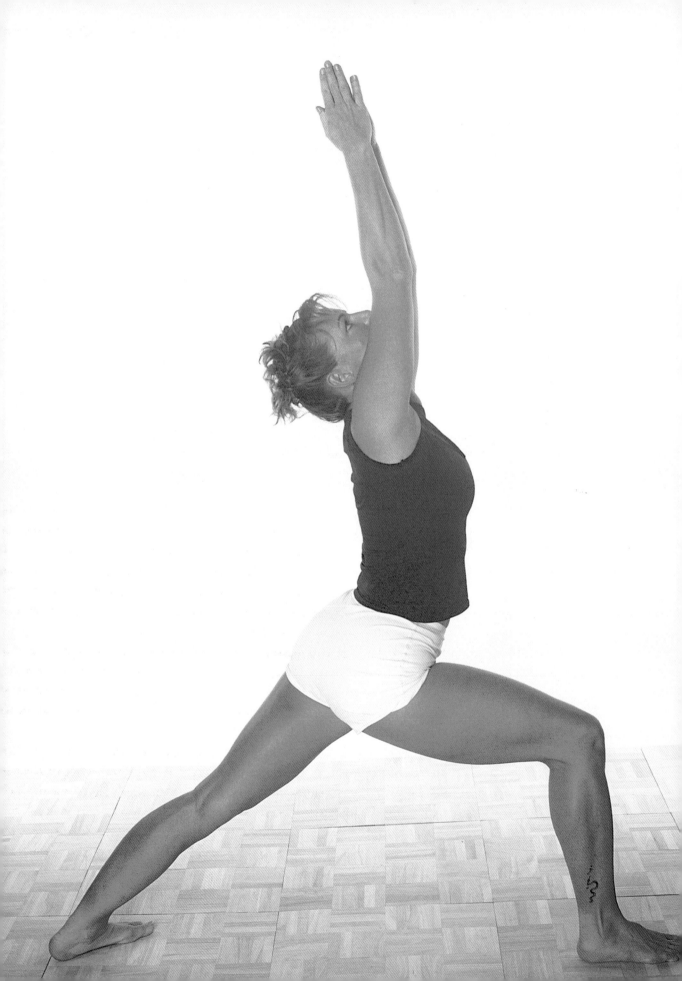

THE WARRIOR SEQUENCE

We complete the Standing Postures with the powerful Warrior Sequence, which builds on the Virabhadrasana posture and incorporates the postures that should by now be familar from the Suryanamaskars A and B.

Remember to focus and move on the breath, stretching as deeply as you can through every asana.

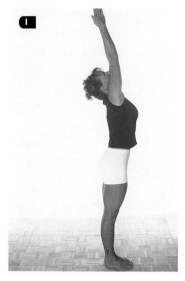
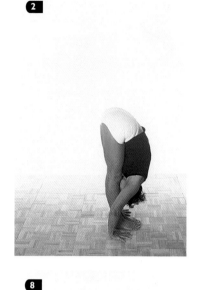
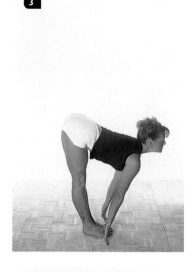

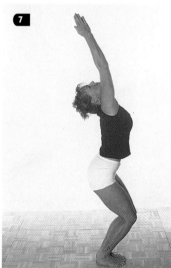
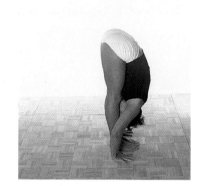
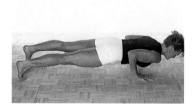

DRISHTI: UPWARDS, HAND, TOES AND NOSE

1. Begin in the posture of Tadasana. Ground your feet, lengthen your spine and draw the crown of your head towards the sky.

2. Inhale and move into Raised Tadasana, reaching up with your arms straight and palms together. Look up at your thumbs (1).

3. Exhale, move into Uttanasana by folding forward from your hips, drop your head and release your spine (2). Inhale, lift your chest and look up (3).

4. Exhale and jump back into Chaturanga Dandasana, the Staff pose (4). If this is too intense, lie down on the mat with your hands by your side-ribs.

5. From the Staff pose, inhale and roll over your toes into Upward Dog. Arch your spine deeply, keeping your legs strong and straight (5).

6. Exhale, roll over your toes into Downward Dog, pushing your hips to the sky. Press your heels into the floor and take one full breath (6).

7. Inhale, bend your knees, look up, and jump straight into Utkatasana (Fierce pose). Drop your pelvis and reach your arms up over your head. Gaze at your thumbs. Hollow your lower belly and lift the root lock. Take five deep Ujjayi breaths (7).

8. Exhale and fold forwards from your hips into Uttanasana, drop your head and release your spine (8). Inhale, lift

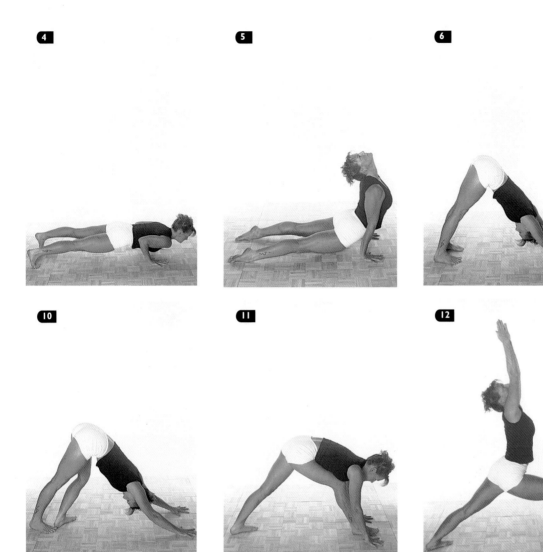

4

5

6

10

11

12

your chest and look up.

9. Exhale and jump back into Chaturanga Dandasana **(9)**. If this is too intense, lie down on the mat with your hands by your side-ribs.

10. Inhale and roll over your toes into the Upward Dog posture, arching your spine and keeping your legs strong and straight.

11. Exhale and roll over your toes into Downward Dog, pushing your hips back. Lower your heels to the floor and take one full breath.

12. Now move in Virabhadrasana A (Right Side). Inhaling, pivot your left heel into your right big toe **(10)**. Place your right foot between your hands and bend deeply into your right thigh, bringing it parallel to the floor **(11)**. Raise your arms over your head, press your palms together and look up. Take five deep Ujjayi breaths **(12)**.

13. Now rotate the posture to face the back of your mat **(13)**. Inhale, straighten your right leg and pivot the ball of your right foot inwards 15

degrees. Exhale and rotate the ball of your left foot outwards 90 degrees. As you do so, rotate your hips to face over your left thigh, drawing your left hip back. Inhale, lift and open your chest and hollow your lower belly. Exhale and bend deeply into your left thigh, bringing it parallel to the floor. Take five deep Ujjayi breaths **(14)**. Be sure to share your weight equally between both legs.

14. From Virabhadrasana A, move onto Virabhadrasana B. Inhale, open

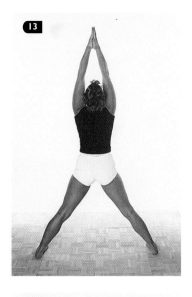

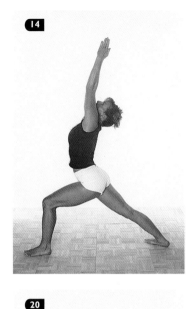

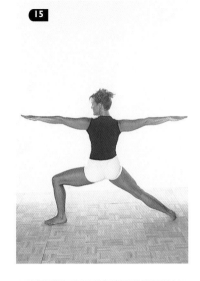

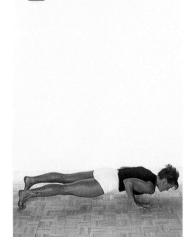

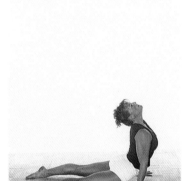

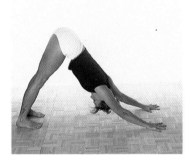

your arms wide, broadening out your collarbones and opening your heart. Draw your right hip back, and open your right shoulder. You are aiming to be as two-dimensional as you can. Lift your upper body out of your pelvis, widening the space between your front hip bones.

Keep your left knee open, stretching your inner left thigh and gaze over your left arm, beyond your fingertips, keeping both arms strong and parallel to the floor. Straighten

your right leg and press your right foot deep into the mat. Share your weight equally between both legs. Take five deep Ujjayi breaths **(15)**.
15. Now rotate Virabhadrasana B to face the front of the mat. Inhale, keeping your arms open wide, straighten your left leg and pivot the ball of your left foot inwards 15 degees. Exhale, rotate the ball of your right foot outwards 90 degrees and bend deep into your right thigh, bringing it parallel to the floor **(16)**.

Draw the left side of your body back, like a bow, and draw your left shoulder away from your left ear. You are aiming to be as two-dimensional as you can. Lift your upper body out of your pelvis, widening the space between your front hip bones.

Keep your right knee open, stretching your inner right thigh and gaze over your right arm, keeping both arms strong and parallel to the floor. Take five deep Ujjayi breaths.
16. Now inhale and bring your left

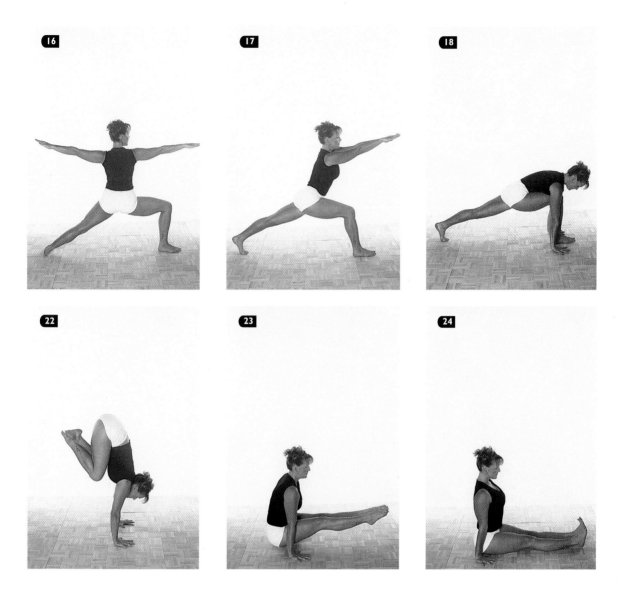

arm around to meet the right, facing the front of your mat. Rotate your hips to face forwards also **(17)**.

17. Exhale, lower your arms, placing your hands beside your front foot **(18)** and step back into Chaturanga Dandasana **(19)**. Empty your lungs.

18. Inhale and roll over your toes into Upward Dog, arching your spine and look up **(20)**.

19. Exhale and then roll over your toes into Downward Dog, pushing

your hips back. Lower your heels to the floor and look towards your navel **(21)**. Take five deep Ujjayi breaths, listening to that sibilant sound like the waves of the sea. Inhale, bend your knees and look up.

20. Inhale, bend your knees, look up and jump your feet **(22 & 23)** between your hands and as you exhale land in the Seated Staff pose **(24)**, The first posture of the Primary Series!

Now we have completed the foundation standing asanas, which, if practised regularly, build inner strength, flexibility and realignment while cultivating a steady, focused mind.

You are now ready to begin the seated postures of the Primary Series which are described in the next chapter.

If you are working with the foundation standing postures only, go to the finishing sequence in Chapter 6 leading towards relaxation.

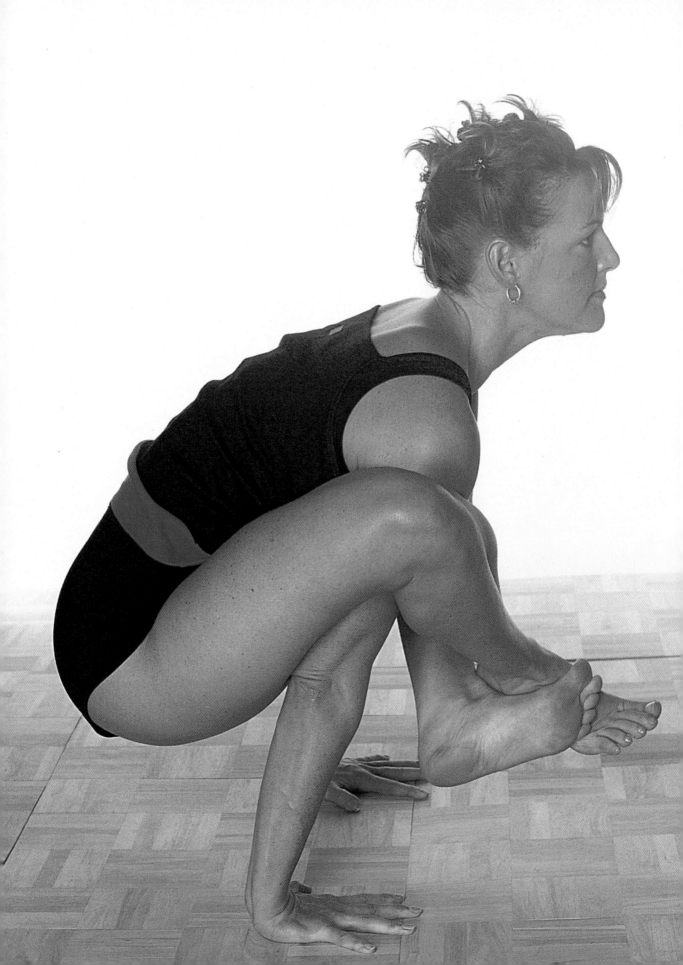

THE PRIMARY SERIES:
SEATED ASANAS

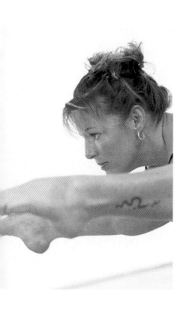

The sequence of standing postures should always be followed by the seated asanas of the Primary Series, which is presented in this chapter. Once you have mastered the Primary Series there are two further series – the Intermediate (or Second) series and the Advanced (or Third) series) – but these are not covered in this book.

Work through this sequence, adding each posture one by one. If you do not complete the series, a good posture with which to close is Navasana, the Boat. When you finish your practice of the Primary Series, go to the Finishing Sequence in Chapter 6, nurturing the body towards relaxation.

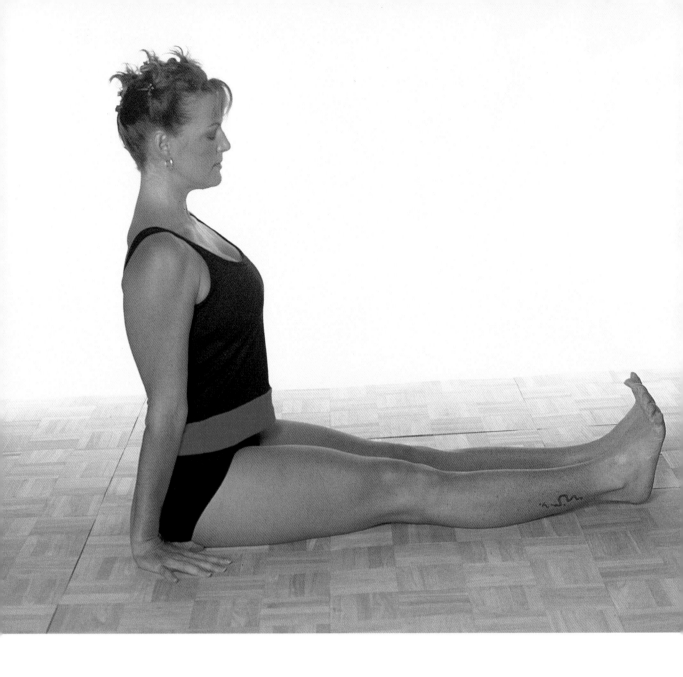

DANDASANA - SEATED STAFF POSE

This is the foundation seated posture and it is very important to "set" the alignment of the body, because this posture dictates the quality of the following sequence.

1. Sitting with your legs extended in front of you, lift the flesh of your buttocks and lengthen your spine.

Press the thoracic spine (the section of spine behind the ribs) between your shoulderblades and lift your front ribs.

2. Roll back your shoulders, broadening across the top chest and collarbones. Lift your ribcage and armpits, softening your shoulders over them.

3. Seal the wall of your abdomen towards your spine and lift the root lock – Mula bandha.

4. Expand your breath into your side-ribs.

5. Take five Ujjayi breaths, focusing on the smooth passageway of air at the back of your throat, creating a sibilant sound. Breathe deeply and mindfully.

PASCHIMOTTANASANA – TUNING THE WEST (BACK) POSE

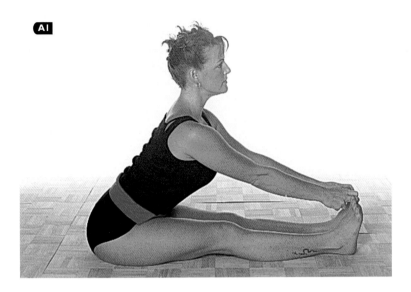

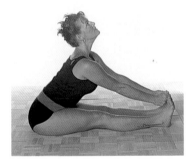

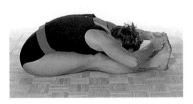

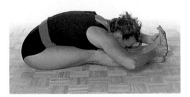

DRISHTI (GAZE POINT):TOES

A

1. Inhale, lift your chest and lengthen your spine. Take five Ujjayi breaths.
2. Exhale and extend your body forwards over your legs, catching your big toes if possible (**A1**).
3. Inhale, lift your chest, look up and hollow your abdomen (**A2**).
4. Exhale and release into the forward bend. Take five Ujjayi breaths.
5. Fold from the front pelvis to help release your lower back (**A3**).

6. Inhale, lift your chest away from your hips, lengthening and hollowing your abdomen and look up. Do not tighten your shoulders or upper body.

B

1. Exhale, fold forwards a little deeper, aiming to catch your feet with your hands (**B1**). Take five Ujjayi breaths.
2. Inhale, lift your chest and look up.
3. Exhale and release the pose.

MODIFICATION:

If you feel a strain in your back, bend your knees, aiming to touch your abdomen on to your thighs; or, hook a belt around your feet. Over time, your lower back will become flexible, and you can straighten your legs.

BENEFITS:

The forward bends of the Primary Series revitalize the abdominal organs and tone the waist, thus improving digestion. The back of the body is intensely stretched, awakening the spine. Forward bends also help to alleviate depression.

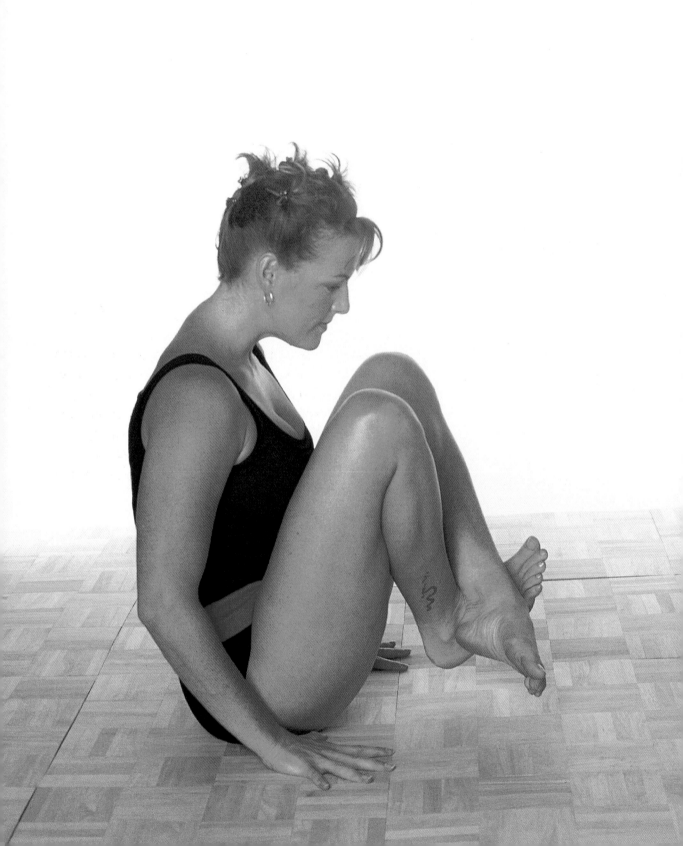

HALF VINYASA

Between every asana, the Half Vinyasa sequence realigns the spine and prepares the body for the next asana, helping to maintain heat and the flow of movement.

Since the Half Vinyasa is partially based on some the poses found in the Suryanamaskars A and B, the sequence is shown here in a similar series of pictures to explain what is involved. You can then refer back to Chapter Four to remind yourself of anything if necessary.

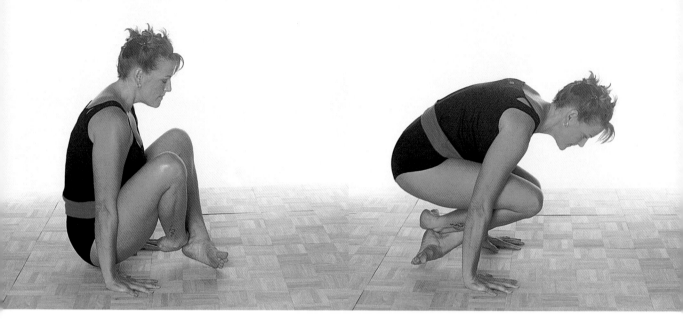

ekam 1 INHALE AND CROSS YOUR LEGS, PLACING YOUR HANDS BESIDE YOUR HIPS. USE THE STRENGTH OF YOUR ARMS TO LIFT YOUR BODY OFF THE FLOOR (THIS MOVEMENT IS CALLED UTH PLUTHI).

due 2 EXHALE AND SWING YOUR LEGS BACK THROUGH YOUR ARMS.

HALF

panca 5 EXHALE, ROLL BACK OVER YOUR TOES INTO DOWNWARD DOG. TAKE ONE FULL UJJAYI BREATH, LENGTHENING YOUR SPINE AND REBALANCING.

sat 6 INHALE, LIFT YOUR HIPS HIGH, BRINGING THEM DIRECTLY ABOVE YOUR SHOULDERS AND HANDS. THIS IS QUITE CHALLENGING, BUT TRY IT! PAUSE FOR A MOMENT, CROSSING YOUR LEGS IN MID-AIR

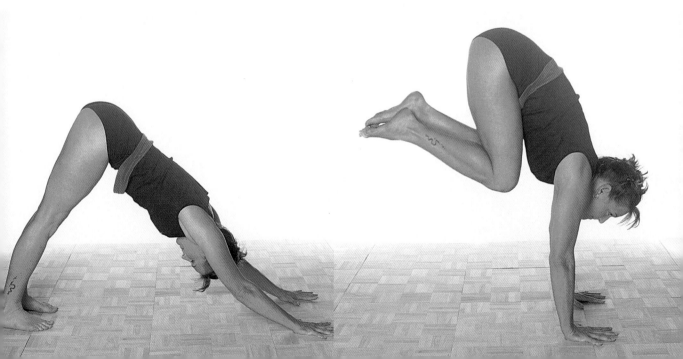

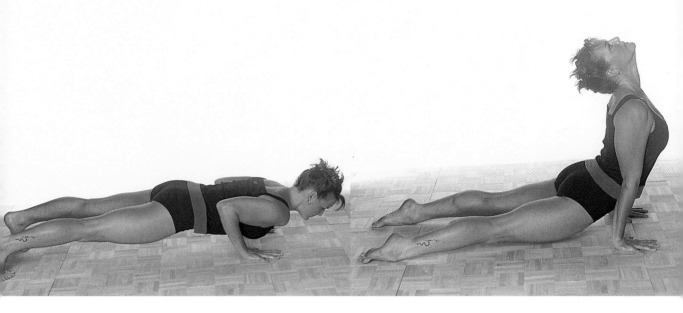

trini 3 LAND IN CHATURANGA, THE STAFF POSE.

catvari 4 INHALE, ROLL OVER YOUR
TOES INTO UPWARD DOG AND LOOK UP.

V I N Y A S A

sapta 7 EXHALE AND SWING YOUR
LEGS THROUGH YOUR ARMS STRETCHING
THEM OUT AS YOU LAND.

astau 8 LAND IN DANDASANA, THE SEATED
STAFF POSE.

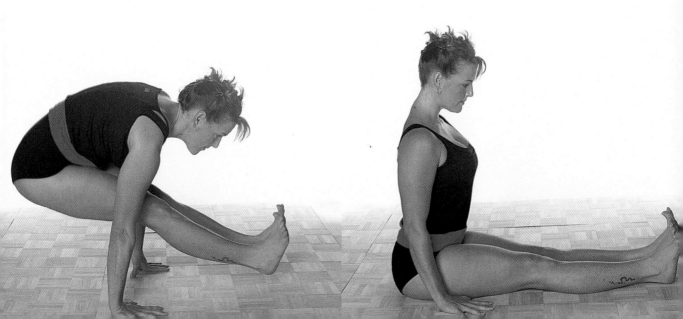

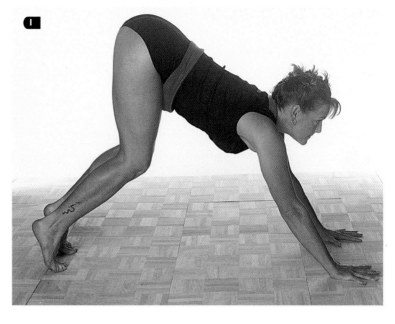

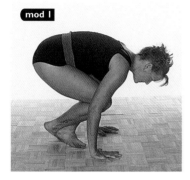

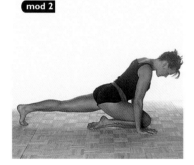

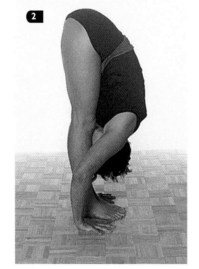

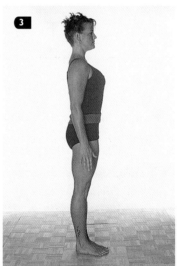

MODIFIED HALF VINYASA

1. Cross your legs, inhale, and roll forwards on to your hands **(mod 1)**.
2. Exhale and jump or step your legs back to Chaturanga **(mod 2)**.
3. Inhale and arch your spine into Upward Dog.
4. Exhale and roll over your toes (or tuck them under) into Downward Dog.
5. Take one full Ujjayi breath, lengthening your spine and rebalancing.
6. Inhale, bend your knees and look up.

7. Exhale, jump your legs up, lifting your hips high and land in a crossed-legged squatting position between your hands. Stretch your legs out in front of you and set Dandasana, the seated Staff pose.

Some practitioners take a full Vinyasa between postures. To do this, repeat the Half Vinyasa as explained through to Downward Dog **(1)**, but instead of jumping

through to the sitting position, jump to Uttanasana **(2)**, then inhale, stand up and move into Tadasana, as if you were completing your Suryanamaskara **(3)**. Then, begin the Suryanamaskara steps 1–6, and when you reach Downward Dog, follow the jump-through to a sitting position. (In other words you will have added a sun-salutation between each posture.)

PURVOTTANASANA – INTENSE EAST ASANA (DIAGONAL PLANK POSE)

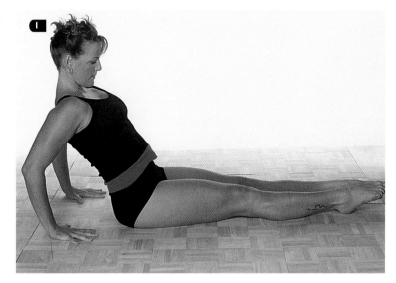

DRISHTI (GAZE POINT): NOSE

1. From Dandasana: exhale, place your hands behind you, fingertips pointing inwards and palms grounded (**1**). Straighten your arms, stretch open your fingers and open your chest. Point your toes.

2. Inhale and raise your hips up, forming a straight angled plank through your body (**2**). Gently drop your head back, without straining your neck (**3**). Seal in the bandhas. Aim to press the balls of your feet and your toes on to the mat.

3. Take five Ujjayi breaths.

4. Exhale, release the pose; inhale and move into Half Vinyasa or the modified Vinyasa.

BENEFITS:

This position counterposes the forward bend, strengthening the heart, waist and spine.

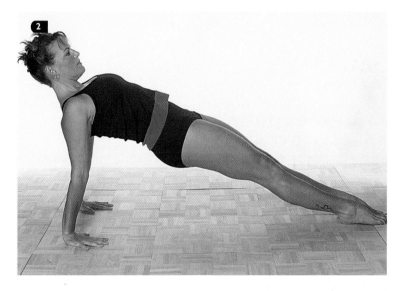

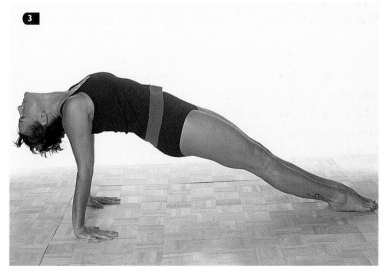

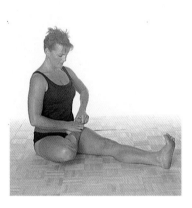

ARDHA BADDHA PADMA PASCHIMOTTANASANA – HALF BOUND LOTUS FORWARD BEND)

DRISHTI (GAZE POINT): TOES

1. From Dandasana: inhale and lift your right leg, bending the knee.
2. Exhale and place your right foot over your left thigh in a half Lotus pose, taking care to rotate your hip and not to strain your knee **(1)**.
3. Inhale, lift and open your chest,
4. Exhale and stretch your body over your extended leg and catch the foot with both hands. **(2)**
5. Press your right heel towards Uddiyana bandha, just below your navel. This is the half Lotus.
6. Face your chest directly over your extended leg, aiming to draw your navel towards your left thigh. Press the back of your left knee down,

sealing the muscles on to the bones of your leg. Flex your left foot, i.e. push your heel away and look up.
7. Take five Ujjayi breaths.
8. Preliminary limber: do not strain your knee. To free your hips, limber by (a) cradling and rocking your right lower leg in your arms; (b) leaning on to your left hand, hold your right foot with your right hand, rocking back and forth.
9. Inhale, look up **(3)**; exhale and release into a forward bend **(4)**.
10. Inhale and move into the Half Vinyasa (see page 92–94).

MODIFICATION:

Do not force yourself into the Lotus. It may develop over years. Look after

your knees. If you feel strain, place your right heel to your groin, dropping your right knee towards the floor.

Full Bound Posture (for advanced practitioners): If you are in a half Lotus, bind your right big toe with your right hand; and your left foot with your left hand.

BENEFITS:

The posture tones abdominal organs and the liver, and alleviates constipation. Healthy blood nourishes the abdomen and genitals, while flexibility increases in the hips, shoulders and back.

2

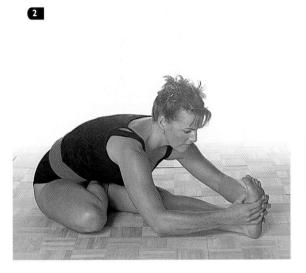

3

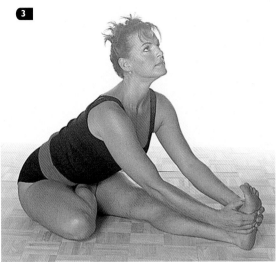

4

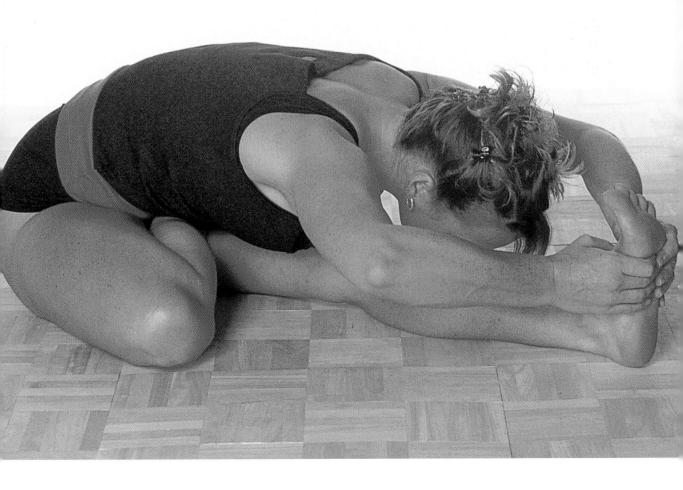

1

2

3

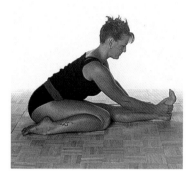

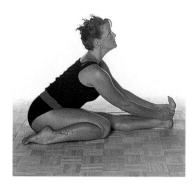

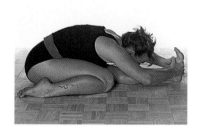

TRIANGMUKHAIKAPADA PASCHIMATTANASANA – THREE (FEET, KNEES AND BUTTOCKS) FACING THE FOOT (INTENSE FORWARD BEND) POSE

DRISHTI (GAZE POINT): TOES

1. From Dandasana, inhale and bend your right knee.
2. Exhale and tuck your lower leg back to a half-kneeling position.
3. Place the top of your right foot on the floor close into your right hip, roll open your calf muscle, and splay the tops of your toes on the floor. Lift the flesh of your right thigh to help ease your right buttock down. Aim to ground both sitting bones, drawing your weight down into your right hip. Hold your left foot with both hands (1).
4. Inhale and lift your chest (2).
5. Exhale and fold your upper body forwards (3)
6. Take five Ujjayi breaths.
7. Align your spine directly over your extended leg.
8. Lift the root lock (the perineum) and hollow your lower belly.
9. Inhale and look up; then exhale and release.
10. Inhale and move into Vinyasa.

Now repeat the posture on the left side.

MODIFICATION:

If necessary, press your left hand into the mat beside you to ease the pressure in your right hip, knee and ankle joints **(mod)**.

BENEFITS:

This posture tones and energizes abdominal organs, frees the ankle joints and improves dropped arches in the feet.

mod

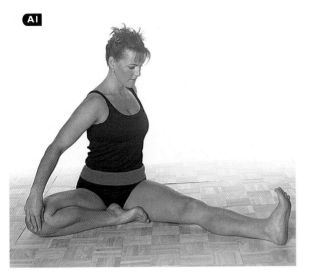

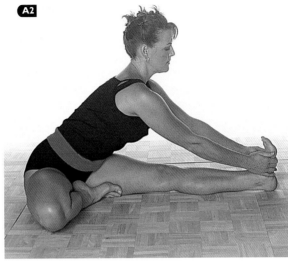

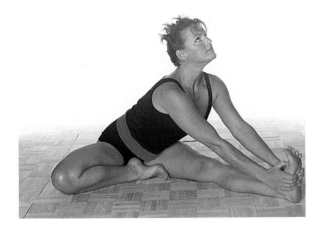

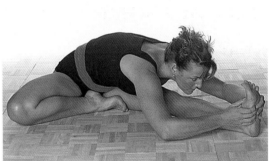

JANU SIRSASANA – HEAD TO KNEE POSE

A

DRISHTI (GAZE POINT): TOES

1. From Dandasana, inhale and place your right heel to the perineum, drawing your right knee up to a 95-degree angle (**A1**).

2. Exhale and face your chest directly over your extended leg.

3. Inhale, open and lift your chest and look up.

4. Exhale and fold forwards, catching your left foot with both hands (**A2**).

5. Inhale, lift the chest, hollow the lower belly and look up (**A3**),

6. Exhale, release and lengthen your spine into a forward bend, aligning the spine over the extended leg. Press the right shoulder down towards the left foot (**A4**).

7. Take five Ujjayi breaths.

8. Inhale and look up; then exhale and release.

9. Inhale and move into Vinyasa.

Now repeat the posture on the left side.

B1

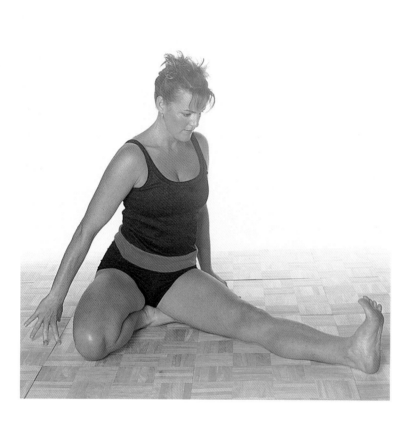

B2

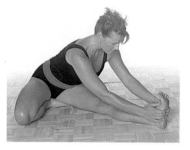

B3

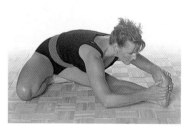

B
DRISHTI (GAZE POINT): TOES

1. From Dandasana, inhale and draw your right heel to your perineum, placing the knee at an 80-degree angle. Exhale and place your hands beside your hips, lifting your hips to sit the perineum on your right heel (your right foot should face towards your left foot) **(B1)**.
2. Align your chest over your extended leg, drawing back your left shoulder.

3. Inhale, lift your chest and look up.
4. Exhale, fold forwards, catching your left foot with both hands **(B2)**.
5. Inhale, lift your chest, hollow the lower belly and look up.
6. Exhale, release and lengthen your spine into a forward bend, aligning your spine over your extended leg **(B3)**. Press your right shoulder down towards the left foot. Now you are sitting on Mula bandha. Take five Ujjayi breaths.
7. Lift the root lock and lengthen your abdomen.

8. Inhale and look up; exhale and release.
9. Inhale and move into Vinyasa.

Now repeat the posture on the left side.

C
DRISHTI (GAZE POINT): TOES

1. From Dandasana, inhale and raise your right foot, holding it with your left hand **(C1)**.

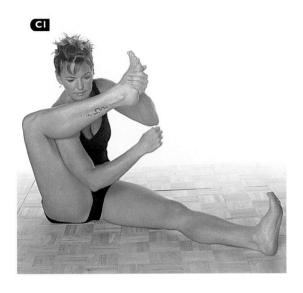

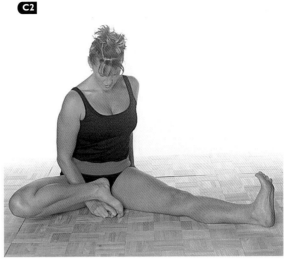

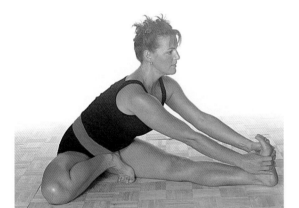

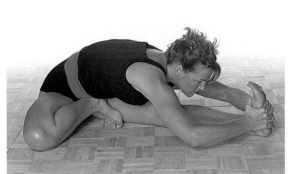

2. Exhale, thread your right arm under your right leg to catch your right toes with your right fingers.

3. Inhale, rotate your foot from the ankle joint, splaying your toes and bringing them to your perineum. Point the heel upwards towards the navel. Aim to lower the right knee towards the floor at a 45-degree angle **(C2)**.

4. Exhale, align your chest over the extended leg, drawing back your left shoulder.

5. Inhale, lift your chest and look up.

6. Exhale and fold forwards, catching your left foot with both hands. **(C3)**

7. Inhale, lift your chest, hollow your lower belly and look up.

8. Exhale, release and lengthen your spine into a forward bend, aligning your spine over your extended leg. Press your right shoulder down towards your left foot **(C4)**. Take five Ujjayi breaths.

9. Inhale and look up; then exhale and release.

10. Inhale and move into Vinyasa.

Now repeat the posture on the left side.

MODIFICATIONS:

Be very careful with your knees! Stay at stage one if necessary, limbering the foot, without attempting to bend the torso forwards.

BENEFITS:

The Janu Sirsasana postures increase flexibility in the lower body. They also cultivate sexual control and balance.

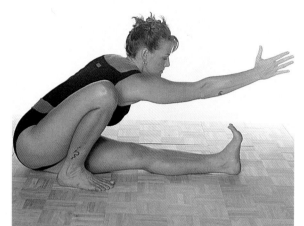

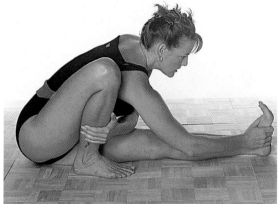

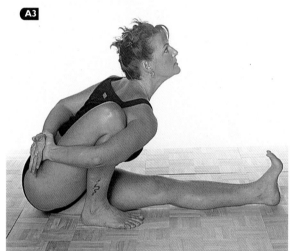

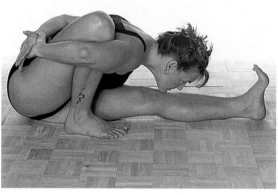

MARICHYASANA SERIES

These four postures are named after the sage Marichi, son of the creator, Brahma.

A
DRISHTI (GAZE POINT): TOES

1. From Dandasana, inhale and bend your right leg to place your right heel in front of your right sitting bone. Keep your foot parallel to your left leg and your right knee raised.

2. Extend your left leg, flexing the foot. Lengthen your spine and lift your chest.
3. Inhale and raise your right arm, lengthening your right waist (**A1**).
4. Exhale and extend your right arm forwards and down, as if to catch the left foot (**A2**). Wrap your right arm around your back, reach your left arm around your back and catch the hands to bind the posture. Aim to hold the left wrist with the right hand.
5. Inhale, lift your chest and look up (**A3**).
6. Exhale, draw your chest to your

left thigh, aiming to touch your chin to your shinbone. Draw your shoulders back and open your chest (**A4**). Take five Ujjayi breaths.
7. Inhale and look up; then exhale and release. Inhale and move into Vinyasa.

Now repeat the posture on the left side.

MODIFICATIONS:
If you strain to bind the pose, stop at stage two and concentrate on your breathing and release into the posture.

B
DRISHTI (GAZE POINT): NOSE

1. From Dandasana, inhale and bend your right leg, pressing your shin bone to your thigh bone.

2. Exhale and place your right foot on the left thigh, in a half Lotus **(B1)**.

3. Inhale and lift your left leg to place the heel in front of the sitting bone. Ground your left foot, and spread your toes **(B2)**.

4. Lengthen your spine and lift your chest. Inhale, raise your left arm up, lengthening the waist and look up **(B3)**.

5. Exhale, and extend your left arm forwards and down, as if to catch the right foot. (It is helpful to draw the shin in tight to the body with the left hand.)

6. Wrap your left arm round your back; and then your right and catch your hands to bind the posture. Aim to hold your left wrist with your right hand. Inhale, lift your chest and look up.

7. Exhale, draw your head to the floor, keeping your shoulders back **(B4)**. Take five Ujjayi breaths.

8. Inhale, lift the chest and look up; then exhale and release the posture.

Now repeat the posture on the left side.

MODIFICATIONS:

Repeat the limber and Lotus modification as given in Ardha Baddha Padma Paschimottanasana (see page 96), placing your left heel to your perineum as in Janu Sirsasana A' (see page 99). Stop at stage two, breathing and releasing into the posture. Practise the posture without the half Lotus.

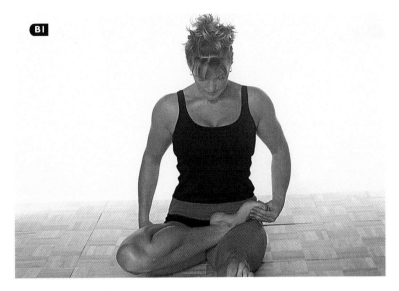

B1

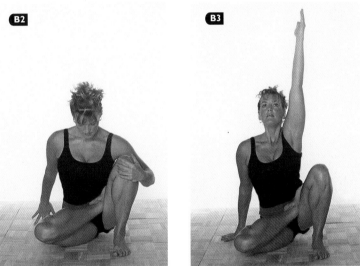

B2

B3

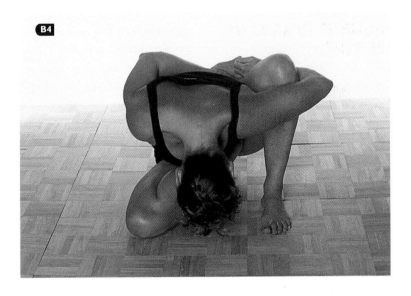

B4

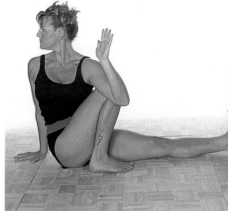

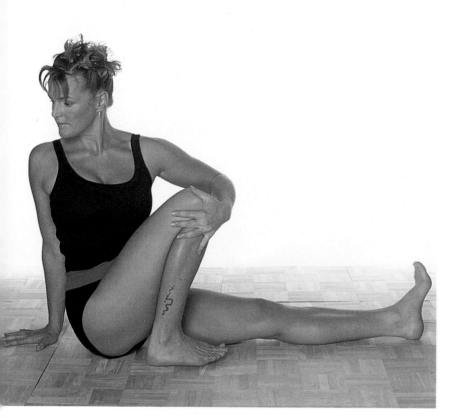

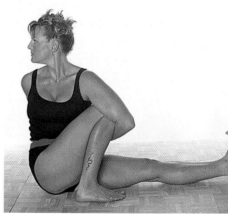

C

DRISHTI (GAZE POINT): FAR LEFT/RIGHT

1. From Dandasana, inhale and lift your right leg, bending it at the knee to place your heel in front of your right sitting bone. Keep your right foot parallel to your left leg. Ground your right foot, and broaden across the ball of the foot, spreading your toes.

2. Exhale and place your right hand behind you, close to the root of your spine, rotating your right shoulder open. Straighten your left leg, flexing the foot (C1).

3. Inhale and raise your left arm, lengthening the waist.

4. Exhale and extend your left arm outside your right thigh, levering your torso into a lateral twist to the right (C2).

5. Inhale and eventually aim to bind the pose by bending your left elbow and wrapping your arm around your thigh, catching both hands behind your back (C3). Aim to hold your right wrist with your left hand (see modification).

6. Take five Ujjayi breaths.

7. Inhale and look to the right; then exhale and release.

8. Inhale and move into Vinyasa.

Now repeat the posture on the left side.

MODIFICATIONS:

Do not force the binding of the pose if you are hunching forwards. Keep your chest open and your shoulders drawn back. Focus on lengthening upwards through the spine as you inhale, and twisting the spine as you exhale.

D
DRISHTI (GAZE POINT): FAR LEFT/RIGHT

1. From Dandasana, inhale and bend your right leg, pressing your shinbone to your thigh bone.

2. Exhale and, rotating from your right hip joint (without straining the knee), place your right foot on your left thigh, in the nook of your hip, in other words moving into a half Lotus (or follow the Modification) **(D1)**.

3. Inhale and bend your left leg to place your heel in front of your left sitting bone **(D2)**. Keep your left foot parallel to your right leg with 6in between the inner edge of your left foot and your right inner thigh. Ground your left foot, and open the ball of the foot, spreading your toes.

4. Exhale and place your left hand behind you, close to the root of your spine, rotating your left shoulder so that it is open. Align your left leg, flexing the foot (you are beginning your spinal twist).

5. Inhale and raise your right arm up, lengthening the waist, and keep looking to the left.

6. Exhale and extend your right arm outside your left thigh, levering your torso into a lateral twist to the left **(D3)**.

7. Inhale and eventually aim to bind the pose by bending your right elbow and wrapping your right arm around your left thigh, catching both hands behind your back. Aim to hold your left wrist with your right hand **(D4)**.

8. Take five Ujjayi breaths.

9. Inhale and look to the left; then exhale and release.

10. Inhale and move into Vinyasa.

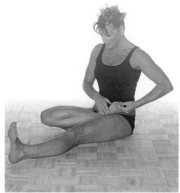

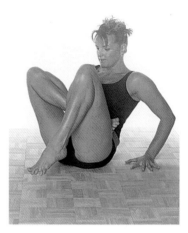

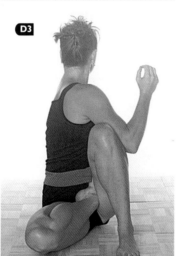

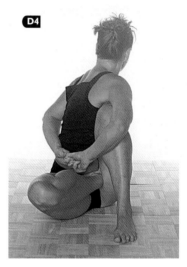

Now repeat the posture on the left side.

MODIFICATIONS:

Inhale and draw your right heel into the perineum. Exhale and lift your left leg, placing the left foot outside the left thigh, keeping the left knee raised. Inhale and hug your left knee with your left arm. Exhale and place your left hand behind you, close to the root of your spine, beginning to twist to the left. Inhale, lengthen your spine and open your chest.

Exhale and deepen the lateral twist to the left, broadening the collarbones. Breathe into your heart.

BENEFITS:

Marichyasana A and B help healthy blood flow to the abdominal organs and spine, while C and D help to relieve pain in the back and hips, as well as opening the shoulders and strengthening the neck. A and B massage the legs and lower back and C and D massage the intestines and aid digestion.

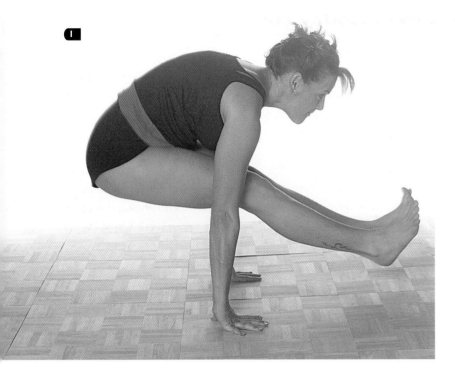

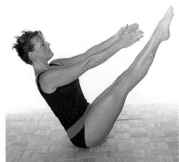

NAVASANA – BOAT POSTURE

DRISHTI (GAZE POINT):
NOSE

1. Advanced practitioners should aim to jump through from Vinyasa without touching their feet to the floor, landing in the following posture **(1)**. Inhale and raise both straight legs to a 45-degree angle, then lean back with your spine straight, balancing on your buttocks.

2. Exhale and stretch out your arms in front of you, pointing your fingertips to your toes. Stretch your legs, pressing them together and squeezing the muscles on to the bones **(2)**.

3. Inhale and lift your chest, breathing into the heart.

4. Exhale and soften your shoulders away from your ears, drawing your navel to your spine.

5. Take five Ujjayi breaths.

6. Exhale and release.

7. Inhale, cross your legs, placing your hands beside your hips and lift up, as in Uth Pluthi, the lift which leads into the half Vinyasa **(3)**.

8. Exhale and repeat Navasana five times, taking five Ujjayi breaths each time. Lift up into Uth Pluthi between each round if possible.

9. After five rounds, exhale and release the posture.

10. Inhale and move into Vinyasa.

MODIFICATIONS:

You can develop the posture in Ardha Navasana, the Half Boat position. As you lean back, hold the backs of your knees with your hands. Bend your knees and find your balance using Uddiyana bandha. Abdominal supports very important to protect and strengthen the lower back. Maintain a straight spine and open your chest, lifting your heart and sternum upwards. Be careful not to press on to your coccyx, the tail of the spine. If this creates any difficulty, use extra padding to protect the coccyx.

BENEFITS:

Navasana tones the waist and nourishes the liver and kidneys. It also strengthens the abdominal muscles and spine.

BHUJAPIDASANA – ARM PRESSURE POSE

DRISHTI (GAZE POINT): NOSE

1. Aim to jump into this posture from the Downward Dog pose in the Vinyasa sequence as follows: from Downward Dog, inhale and jump your legs around your arms (as if leap-frogging around them). Bring the backs of your knees as high as possible, around your shoulders **(1)**.

2. Exhale and squeeze your thighs around your shoulders, keeping your palms grounded and your fingers stretched open.

3. Inhale and rest your inner thighs on the outside edges of the upper arms (as if they were ledges). Find your balance.

4. Exhale and gently lift your feet off the floor – aim to interlock your feet together in front of you. If you can't do this, start by touching your big toes together.

5. At first you may have to bend your elbows, but with practice, aim to straighten your arms and look forwards **(2)**.

6. Balance on your arms, and take five Ujjayi breaths.

7. Move into the advanced full posture by exhaling, then lower your head or chin to touch the floor in front of you **(3)**. Take five Ujjayi breaths.

8. Now move into Bakasana (the Crane posture) by inhaling, then coming up and bringing your legs around to balance your knees on the backs of your arms **(4)**. Take one Ujjayi breath.

9. Exhale and jump back into Chaturanga Dandasana, the Staff posture (if you are an advanced practitioner). Alternatively, step back to prepare your Vinyasa.

MODIFICATIONS:

Just practise as far as you can, breathing deeply. You may need to remain at stage one. Keeping your hips high, hold the backs of your ankles with your hands, and work your shoulders through your legs. Enjoy! A squatting position is a good alternative posture to limber open the hips.

BENEFITS:

The arm balances develop upper body strength, toning the shoulders, arms and waist. Lightness in the body is cultivated as one learns to harness the bandhas while the oesophagus is purified.

1

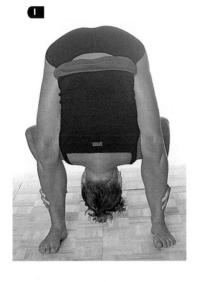

2

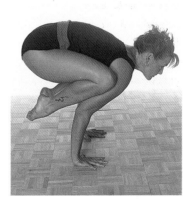

3

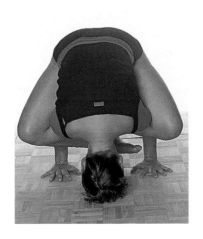

4

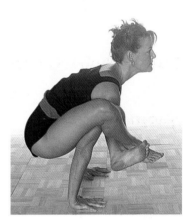

KURMASANA – RECLINING TORTOISE POSE

DRISHTI (GAZE POINT): THIRD EYE

1. Once again, aim to jump from the Downward Dog pose into this posture, as in Bhujapidasana (see page 107). From Downward Dog, inhale and jump (as if leap-frogging) your legs around your arms, bringing the backs of your knees as high as possible, around your shoulders (1).

2. Exhale and squeeze your thighs around your shoulders as much as you can.

3. Inhale and rest your thighs on the ledges of your upper arms, balancing the left and right sides of your body.

4. Exhale and gently lower your hips to the floor, using the strength of your arms (2).

5. Inhale, extend your arms wide under your thighs, with your palms facing down; then stretch your legs out wide in front of you as straight as possible.

6. Exhale and release into the posture, drawing your chest and chin to the floor. Flex your feet (3).

7. Take five Ujjayi breaths. It is recommended that you try to stay in Kurmasana for up to 30 breaths to deepen it.

8. Inhale and look up; then exhale and release gently.

9. Inhale and move into Vinyasa, or go straight into Supta Kurmasana.

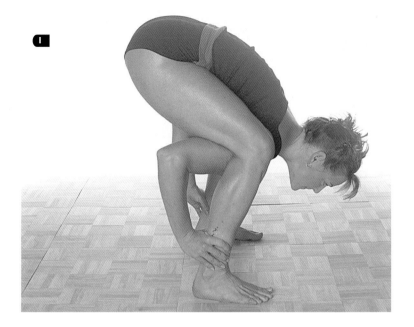

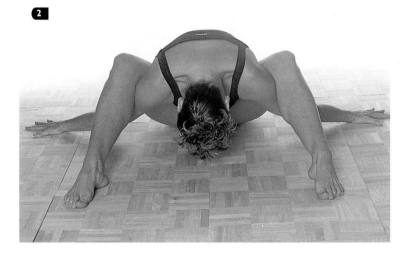

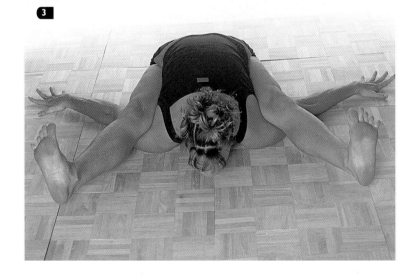

SUPTA KURMASANA – SLEEPING TORTOISE POSE

This is an advanced position and should be learnt only with the aid of an experienced teacher who can help to adjust your alignment. Don't be disheartened if it takes time, as it is a serious posture! The final stage of the asana resembles a tortoise withdrawn inside its shell, symbolizing pratyahara – sense-withdrawal from the outside world.

DRISHTI (GAZE POINT): THIRD EYE

1. With arms and legs straight and your chest and chin bent towards the floor in front of you in Kurmasana (see opposite), inhale and bend your elbows, wrapping your arms behind your back **(1)**.
2. Exhale and clasp your hands together, binding the posture **(2)**.
3. Inhale and place your left foot behind your head.
4. Exhale and place your right foot over your head, interlocking the feet.
5. Take five Ujjayi breaths **(3)**.
6. Releasing your hands, press them into the mat beside your hips, fingertips facing forwards.
7. Inhale and using the strength of your arms, lift your body up, and look up **(4)**. Advanced practitioners should aim to maintain their legs behind their head.
8. Take five Ujjayi breaths.
9. Release the posture in the same manner as Bhujapidasana, via

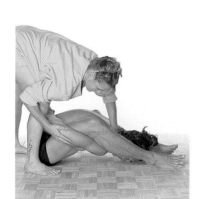

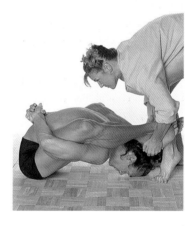

Bakasana (the Crane posture) for one breath, jumping the legs back into Vinyasa on the exhale.
10. Move into Vinyasa.

MODIFICATIONS:

Begin the practice from a seated position, stretching your legs out wide. Aim to thread your arms under your legs, stretching them out also and lower your torso towards the floor in front of you. Protect your body with the bandhas, drawing your abdomen back, and keep breathing, deeply and freely.

BENEFITS:

A sacred posture, Supta Kurmasana draws the senses inwards and focuses the mind, preparing the body for the higher limbs of yoga. It purifies the lungs, heart, root of the nervous system and abdominal organs as well as toning the spine. The effects are as if awakening from a deep sleep.

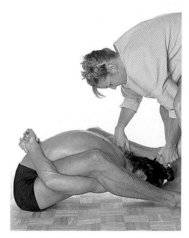

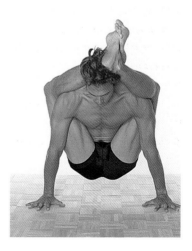

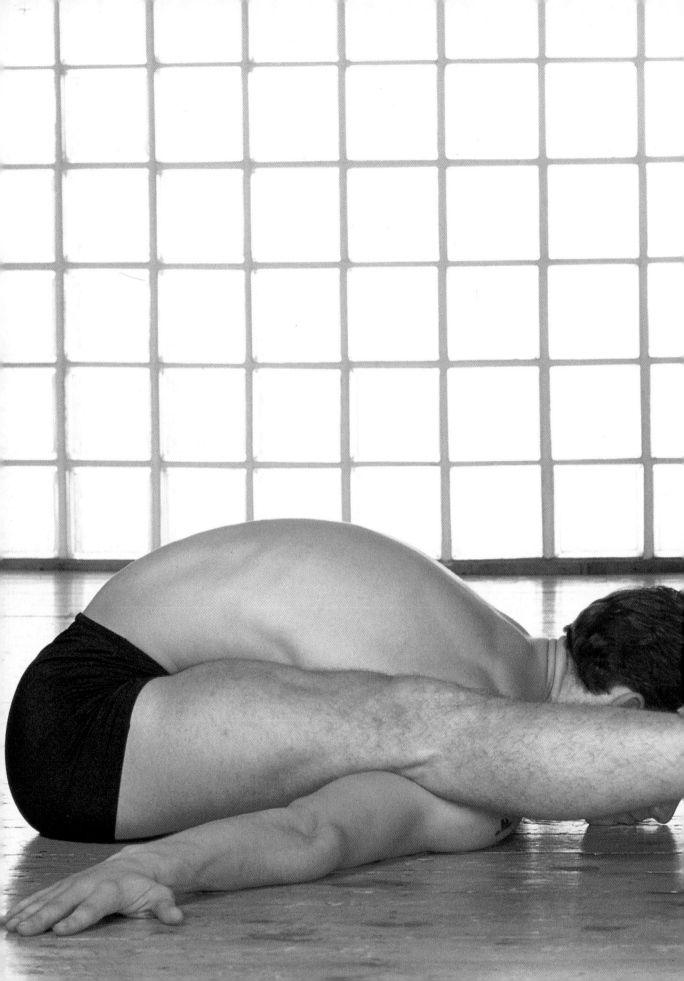

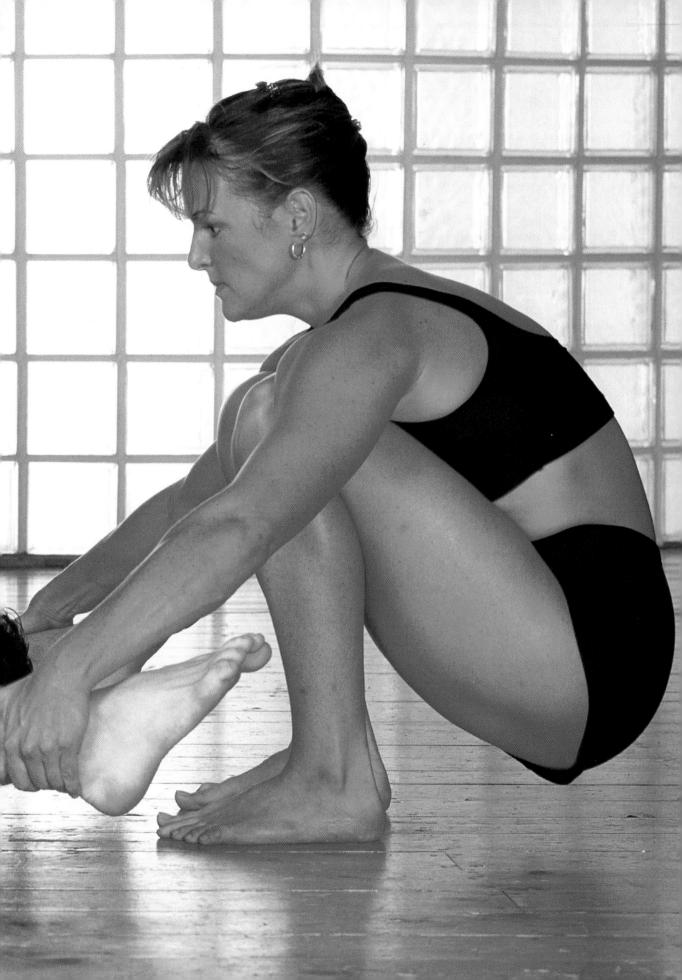

GARBHA PINDASANA – EMBRYO IN THE WOMB POSE

Again, this is an advanced position which should only be attempted under the supervision of a teacher. Make sure you have a padded mat to protect your spine as you will be rocking backwards and forwards.

DRISHTI (GAZE POINT): NOSE

1. From Dandasana, inhale and draw your right foot into the half Lotus **(1)**.
2. Exhale and draw your left foot on top of your right thigh **(2)**. You are now in a full Lotus posture.
3. Inhale and work your hands through the space between your thighs and calf muscles **(3)**. Keep breathing, working your arms through until your elbows can be bent to cup your face with your hands together.
4. Inhale and prepare to roll your body back on to the mat **(4)**.
5. Exhale and rock your body back on your spine **(5)**.
6. Inhale and roll up into a sitting position **(6)**.
7. Exhale and rock your body back on to your spine.
8. Inhale and again roll up into a sitting position.
9. Repeat this rocking movement (i.e. steps 7 and 8) nine times, until you have taken nine Ujjayi breaths in total. This signifies the nine months of gestation.

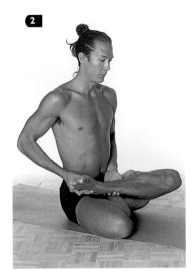

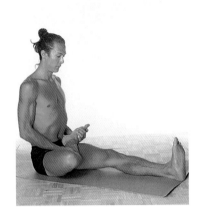

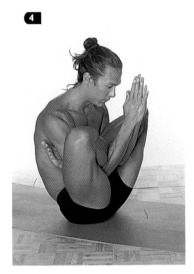

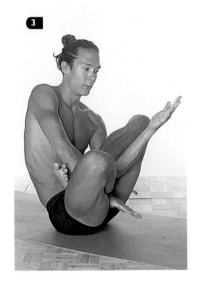

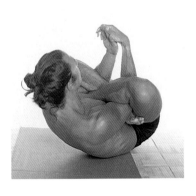

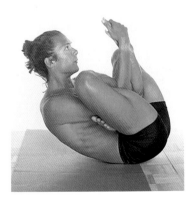

KUKKUTASANA – COCK POSE

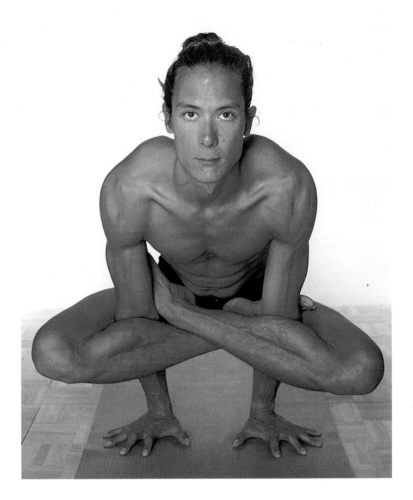

This is another advanced posture, requiring much Uddiyana bandha control and follows straight on from the previous posture.

DRISHTI (GAZE POINT): NOSE

1. On the tenth inhale after Garbha Pindasana, roll your body up into a sitting position.
2. Press your hands deep into the mat with your fingers spread wide and lift your hips.
3. Balance for five Ujjayi breaths.
4. Inhale and look up; then exhale and release.
5. Inhale and move into Vinyasa.

MODIFICATIONS:

The advanced nature of the two previous postures requires working with a teacher. Limber your hips as in Ardha Baddha Padma Paschimottanasana (see page 96). Practise sitting in a half Lotus, changing legs after 10 breaths each side, or just sit cross-legged, keeping your spine straight, and practise your breathing awareness and bandha control.

BENEFITS:

These postures help strengthen the spine, abdomen and wrists. Blood flows to the abdominal organs, purifying the liver and the intestines.

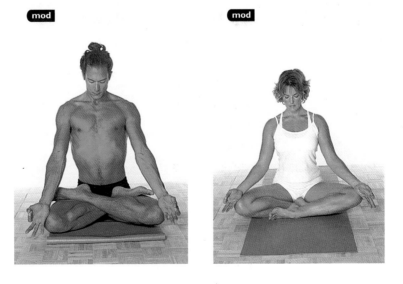

BADDHA KONASANA – BOUND ANGLE POSE

DRISHTI (GAZE POINT): NOSE

1. From Dandasana, sitting with your spine lengthened, inhale, bend your knees and catch your feet, opening your hips like a butterfly's wings.
2. Exhale and gather your heels into your perineum, pressing your hips towards the floor **(1)**.
3. Inhale and lift and broaden your chest, opening your collarbones.

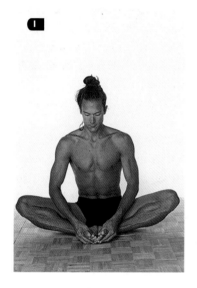

Clarify the bandhas.
4. Exhale and, if you are an advanced practitioner, open the soles of your feet to face upwards, like a book **(2)**.
5. Inhale, lift your chest and look up, hollowing your lower belly.
6. Exhale and lower your torso forwards from the sacrum and hips. Continue to move forwards with every breath, drawing chest and chin to the floor **(3)**. Take five Ujjayi breaths.
7. Inhale, lift your chest and look up, hollowing your lower belly.
8. Exhale and curl your head inwards to place your brow on the soles of your feet. Take five Ujjayi breaths.
9. Inhale and look up; then exhale and release.
10. Inhale and move into Vinyasa.

MODIFICATIONS:

Work to the maximum of your ability and remember to keep breathing deeply. Do not force the forward bend from the upper body. Relax your shoulders and initiate the movement from your hips. Soften the brain, i.e. don't strain, but relax your eyes and the space behind them. Focus on the sound of your breathing, like the waves of the sea.
If it is too difficult to bend forwards, limber by pressing your palms behind you, lift your chest, lean back and take five Ujjayi breaths. Press your knees down towards the floor. Alternate, forwards and backwards, working to open the hips and move from the core of your body, supporting your lower back with the Uddiyana bandha lift.

BENEFITS:

The increased blood flow cleanses the pelvic region, abdomen and back, especially nourishing the kidneys and the bladder. The posture also helps to avoid varicose veins, as well as regulate the menstrual cycle. It is excellent for constipation and indigestion.

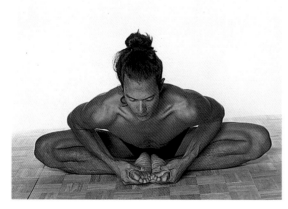

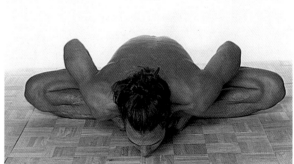

UPAVISTHA KONASANA – EXTENDED ANGLE POSE

DRISHTI (GAZE POINT): THIRD EYE

1. From Dandasana, inhale and stretch your legs wide, flexing your feet, i.e. pushing the heels away.
2. Exhale and lift the flesh of your buttocks to sit on the front of the sitting bones.
3. Inhale, lengthen your spine, lift and open the chest and look up **(1)**.
4. Exhale and fold into a forward bend, catching your feet with your hands. Aim to press your thumb between the first and second long bones (below the first and second toes) and wrap your fingers around the outside edges of your feet.
5. Inhale, lift your chest and look up.
6. Exhale and draw your chest and chin to the floor, lengthening your spine out of the sacrum. Seal in the lower locks to cultivate core strength and keep your legs strong and straight **(2)**.
7. Take five Ujjayi breaths.
8. Inhale, lift your chest and look up. Open your arms wide, and lift your feet up into your hands, balancing on your buttocks **(3)**. Advanced practitioners should aim to raise the body up while still holding the feet. This is extremely difficult though!
9. Take another five Ujjayi breaths.
10. Inhale and look up; then exhale and release.
11. Inhale and move into Vinyasa.

MODIFICATIONS:

Practise the balance from a seated position, bending your knees to catch your feet. Gently lean back, aiming to lift your heart and chest as much as you can. Gradually straighten your legs. Harness Uddiyana bandha and keep breathing.

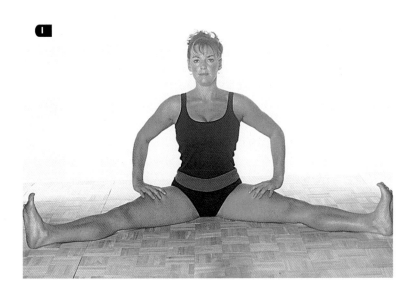

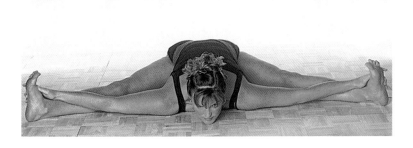

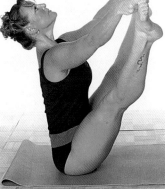

SUPTA KONASANA – SUPINE ANGLE POSE

Make sure you have a padded mat to protect your spine. We are repeating the same posture, this time balancing on the shoulders in an inverted position and swinging through to a forward bend.

DRISHTI (GAZE POINT): NOSE

1. From Dandasana, inhale and swing your legs over your head, balancing on your shoulders. Pay attention to your neck – don't press on the neck vertebrae (1).
2. Exhale, hook your fingers round your toes and lengthen your spine, drawing your navel inwards. Move your outstretched legs wide apart (2).
3. Inhale and swing your body up to balance on your buttocks, finding your balance, maintaining the outstretched legs and pointing your toes. Look up, open the chest and pause on the full inhalation (3).
4. Exhale and gently allow your body to fold forwards into a seated forward bend, maintaining the outstretched legs throughout the sequence (4).
5. Inhale, lift the chest and look up.
6. Exhale and release the posture.
7. Inhale and move into Vinyasa.

MODIFICATIONS:

Practise each stage of the posture separately, working as deeply as you can. Don't strain your body (particularly your spine – make sure your mat is folded to provide adequate padding), but focus on the movement of the breath washing through your body.

BENEFITS:

The two previous asanas help to tone the abdomen and legs, as well as helping to broaden the chest and shoulders. They stretch the hamstrings and strengthen the spine.

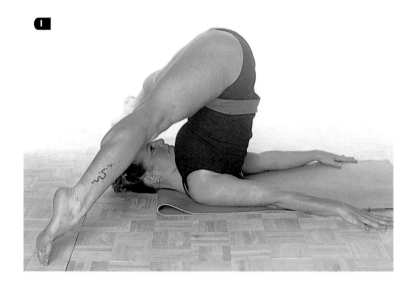

1

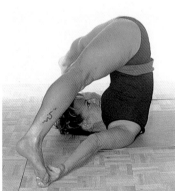

2

3

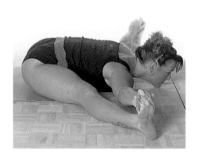

4

SUPTA PADANGUSTHASANA – SUPINE FOOT-TOE POSE, OR LEG RAISES

DRISHTI (GAZE POINT): TOES, FAR LEFT/RIGHT

1. From Dandasana, lie flat and lengthen your spine. Broaden across your shoulders and chest to balance the left and right sides of your body **(1)**.
2. Inhale and raise your right leg straight, hooking your big toe with your right hand **(2)**. Press your left hand on to your left thigh, to keep your left leg straight, and point your toes.
3. Exhale and raise your chin to your right shin, lifting your trunk off the floor using the strength of Uddiyana bandha. Take five Ujjayi breaths.
4. Inhale and place your head back on the floor, keeping the neck lengthened.
5. Exhale and take your leg wide to the right, aiming to place the leg on the floor, with the foot parallel to your right ear. Turn your head to gaze over your left shoulder **(3)**.

Try to keep your left hip and left shoulder pressed down into the mat and press the backs of both shoulders and hips to the floor. Take five Ujjayi breaths.
6. Inhale, return your leg to the centre and catch your foot with both hands, touching your chin to the shin **(4)**.
7. Exhale, lay your head down again, lengthen the back of your neck and draw your right foot towards your right ear. Take five Ujjayi breaths.
8. Exhale, release your right leg and change sides.

Now repeat the posture on the left side.

MODIFICATIONS:

If you cannot catch the foot of the raised leg, bend your knee and hold your shin instead (mod on page 118). Don't strain your lower back or hips. Check you are centred and lengthen your spine. Initiate your movements from the spine and the lower locks, cultivating core strength. Do not throw yourself off-balance. Be sure to keep your shoulders open and your neck released.

To limber, hug your thighs into your body and rock sideways to release your lower back, hips and neck, gently rolling your head from side to side.

BENEFITS:

This deep stretch for the legs cleanses and opens the pelvic region, circulating healthy blood to the hips and legs. The waist is toned and Uddiyana bandha is developed, cultivating lightness.

Having completed both sides, either move into the following position – Chakorasana (the Wheel) – and from there into Vinyasa or, if you have a weak neck, omit Chakorasana and move straight into Vinyasa. You should learn Chakorasana with the supervision of a teacher.

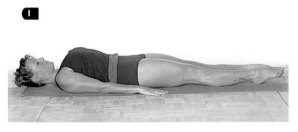

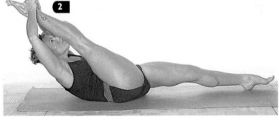

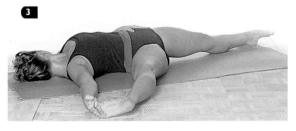

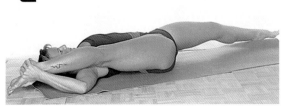

mod

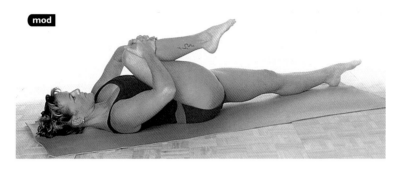

1

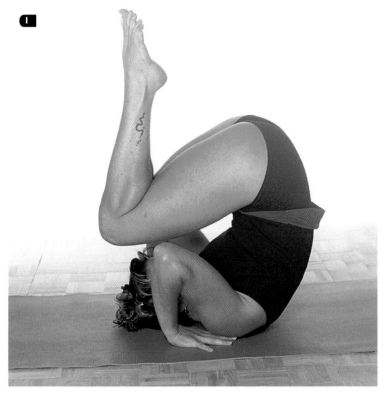

2

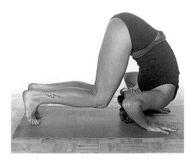

CHAKORASANA – WHEEL POSE

1. Inhale and press your palms beside your ears.

2. Exhale and prepare your body to roll over, harnessing the bandhas.

3. Inhale and swing your legs over your head, bending your knees into a backward roll (**1**, **2**, **3**).

4. Exhale and land in Chaturanga Dandasana, the Staff pose, if possible, ready to move into Vinyasa.

MODIFICATIONS:

You can omit the wheel and simply hug your thighs into your abdomen to limber up your hips and sacrum, rocking gently on your back.

3

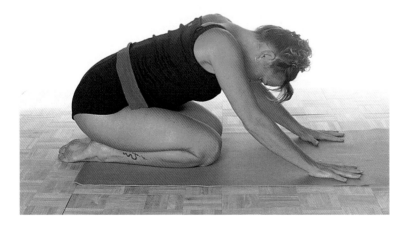

UBHAYA PADANGUSTHASANA – BOTH BIG TOES POSE

You will need a padded mat to protect the spine for this posture. Anyone who has a neck problem should practise the Modification for this pose.

BENEFITS:

This posture helps to purify the whole pelvic region, as well as toning the waist and stomach.

DRISHTI (GAZE POINT): NOSE

1. From Dandasana, lie flat on your mat.

2. Inhale and swing your legs over your head, balancing on your shoulders.

3. Exhale, hook your toes with your fingers and lengthen your spine, drawing your navel inwards and squeezing the inner seams of your legs together (1).

4. Inhale and swing your body up to balance on your buttocks, finding your balance (2).

5. Exhale and gently drop your head back, looking up. Hang from your toes (3).

6. Take five Ujjayi breaths.

7. Inhale and look up; then exhale and release.

8. Inhale and move into Vinyasa.

MODIFICATIONS:

If you have neck problems, enter the posture from a seated position, bending your knees and catching your toes. Gradually straighten your legs. Keep your spine as straight as possible, lifting your chest and softening your shoulders. Move from your centre in the lower belly.

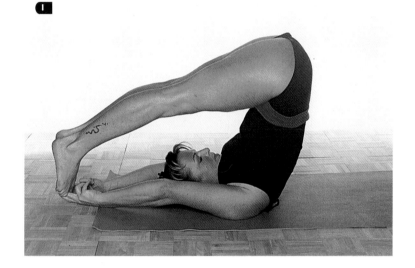

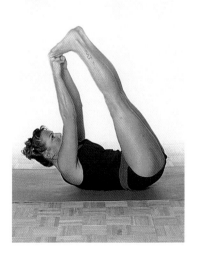

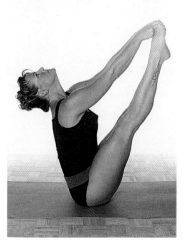

URDHVA MUKHA PASCHIMOTTANASANA – HALF FACE FORWARD BEND POSE

Use a padded mat for this position to protect your spine. Fold your yoga mat in two so that when you roll on your spine it has a soft surface beneath it.

DRISHTI (GAZE POINT): TOES

1. From Dandasana, inhale and swing your legs over your head, balancing on your shoulders. Be sensitive to any pressure on the neck vertebrae.

2. Exhale and take hold of the outside edges of your feet and squeeze the inner seams of your legs together. Lengthen your spine, drawing your navel inwards. Don't strain your neck.

3. Inhale and swing your body up to balance on your buttocks, finding your balance.

4. Exhale and aim to sandwich your body into a deep forward bend, while still balancing on your buttocks. Draw your abdomen towards your thighs and your face to your knees. Look up towards your big toes (1).

5. Take five Ujjayi breaths.

6. Inhale and look up; then exhale and release.

7. Inhale and move into Vinyasa.

MODIFICATIONS:

It is difficult to hold the feet and manage to swing up to this seated balance. Instead, hold your ankles or calves and cultivate your balance (mod). Repeat the modification suggested for the previous posture, aiming to hold your feet.

Practise the modification until you have developed the posture with an experienced teacher.

BENEFITS:

This posture helps healthy blood flow to the head and nourish the lower back, oesophagus and pelvic region. A feeling of lightness is cultivated as the lower bandhas are practised.

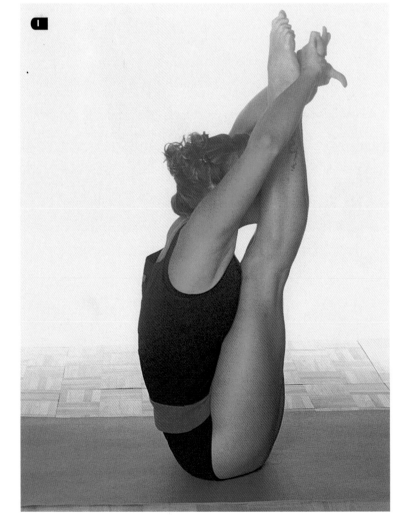

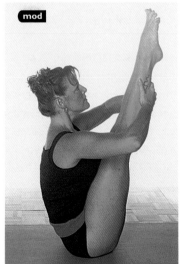

SETU BANDHASANA – FORMING A BRIDGE POSE

DRISHTI (GAZE POINT): NOSE

1. From Dandasana, inhale and bend your knees, drawing your heels together. Splay the feet wide like Charlie Chaplin, spreading your toes and pressing the balls of your feet into the mat **(1)**.
2. Exhale and measure two hands' distance between your heels and perineum. Continue to breathe as you set the posture. (Eventually, when you lift up your hips into the full posture, your hips should be raised and your legs straight.)
3. Exhale and lean back on to your elbows, lifting your chest high, and gently drop your head back **(2)**.
4. (For advanced practitioners only.) Inhale and place the crown of your head on the mat. Your spine should be arched but your hips remain on the mat **(3)**.
5. Exhale and prepare to lift yourself up.
6. Inhale and raise your hips up, lifting your bodyweight on to the crown of your head.
7. Keep your feet grounded and the balls of your feet pressed down.
8. Straighten your legs as much as you can. Bring your arms across your chest, drawing your shoulders back. Roll right up on to the crown of your head **(4)**.
9. Take five Ujjayi breaths.
10. Exhale and gently release yourself down, lengthening out the back of your neck.

11. Move into Chakorasana (see page 118) and from there into Vinyasa.

MODIFICATIONS:
Only practise this when you have had tuition with a teacher, as it causes intense pressure on the neck. Set your feet and legs in the same manner. Lie down on the mat, lengthening your spine.

Soften and widen your shoulders, and release the back of your neck. Inhale and raise your hips, drawing your navel to your spine and lifting the root lock. Take five Ujjayi breaths. Exhale and gently release your body down, uncurling the spine like a fern. To limber, hug your thighs into your body and rock sideways to release your lower back and hips. Then move into Vinyasa.

BENEFITS:
Setu Bandhasana helps to tone and cleanse the heart, lungs and oesophagus, as well as the waist and neck. It also purifies the pelvic region and stimulates your digestion.

You have now completed the Primary Series of Seated Asanas and can move on to the Finishing Sequence in the next chapter.

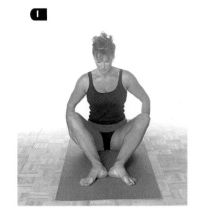
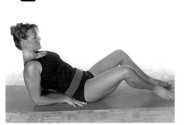
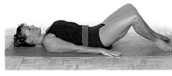
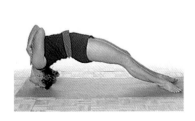

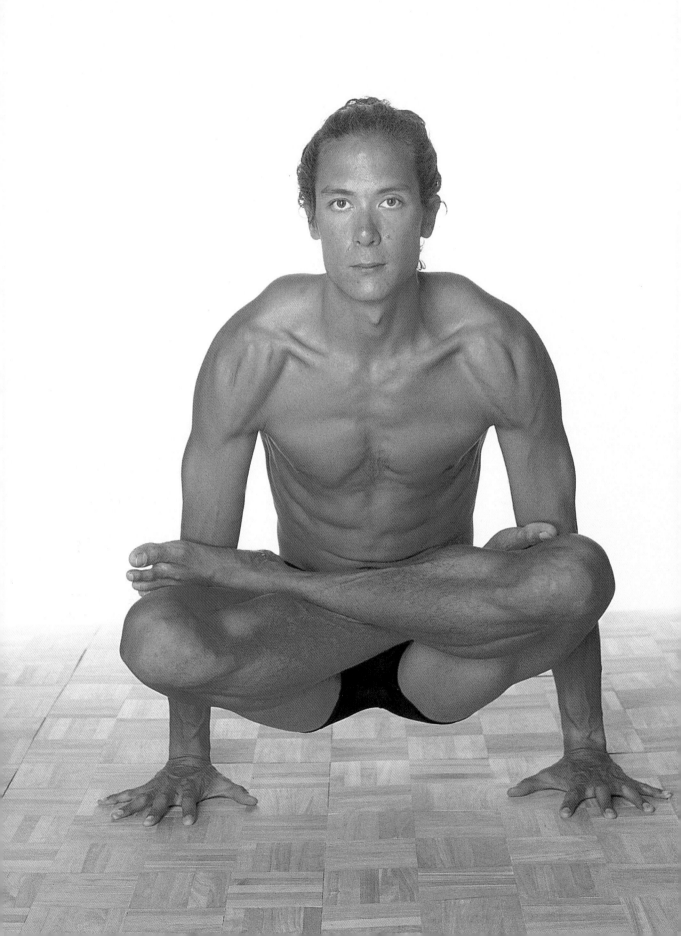

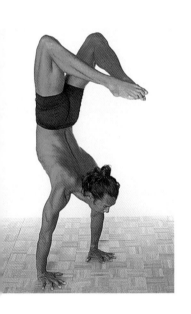

THE FINISHING SEQUENCE – NURTURING THE BODY TOWARDS RELAXATION

The Finishing Sequence in Astanga Yoga includes the inverted postures of the shoulderstand and headstand and the sitting breathing practice which culminates in deep relaxation. We practise backbends at this stage and introduce handstand work to develop upper body strength and balance. The final inversions soothe the body and give tremendous benefits, but must be learnt carefully with a teacher so as to avoid pressure on the neck.

URDHVA MUKHA VRKSASANA – UPWARD-FACING TREE – HANDSTAND PRACTICE

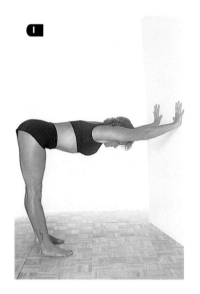

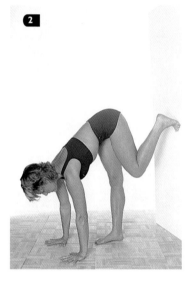

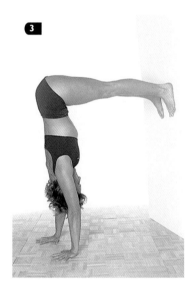

You should only practise this under the guidance of a teacher.

HALF HANDSTAND

(Optional)

Preparation using wall.

1. Place your palms on the wall in a forward bend **(1)**.

2. Straighten your spine, parallel to the floor, and charge your legs, i.e. press the muscles on to the bones. Place your feet hip-width apart. This is good alignment practice for

Downward Dog.

3. Lengthen your arms, lift your front ribs away from your pelvis and draw your navel towards your spine, hollowing the lower belly.

4. Dig your thoracic spine, i.e. the section of the spine behind the ribs, between your shoulderblades.

5. Now invert the posture by placing your hands into your footprints and then walking your feet up the wall to where your hands were **(2)**. Lift your hips and apply exactly the same principles of alignment. You should try to

make your arms strong, like pillars **(3)**.

7. Look at a spot between your hands, about six inches in front of them.

8. Work up to 30 breaths. Rest when necessary. Keep your palms wide and your fingers spread, and push the floor away from you.

9. To recover, rest in a soft standing forward bend to release your spine and ease out your shoulders, or rest in the Child's Pose (see page 140).

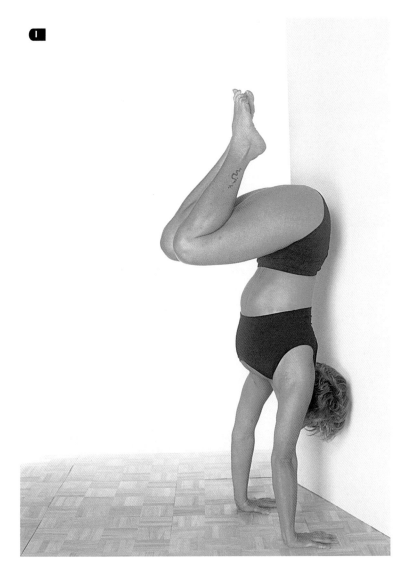

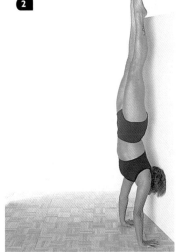

FULL HANDSTAND

Don't run and jump into the handstand! This is a controlled lift, using the support of the bandhas and the steady strength of the arms. Instead, bunny-hop, using the wall.

1. Place your hands shoulder-width apart, with your fingertips six inches away from the wall. Look at a point just in front of you, on the floor.
2. Place your feet together, lifting your hips high.

3. Inhale, bend your knees and bunny-hop your hips up, directly above your hands **(1)**.
4. Like a pendulum motion, lift up the pelvis on the inhale, and straighten you legs. Pause (if you can) for a moment in mid-air, clarifying Uddiyana bandha to cultivate balance **(2)**.
5. Exhale, come down, landing gently with soft knees.
6. Keep practising.

This breaks down the handstand into sections. Try to hinge at the hips, holding Uddiyana bandha firmly to support the lower back. Your arms, spine and hips should be in a straight line. Then straighten your legs. The wall will stop you from falling over. Advanced practitioners may work on lifting the legs off the floor without needing to jump, due to the strength in the Uddiyana bandha. But this requires a lot of practice.

URDHVA DHANURASANA – UPWARD FACING BOW

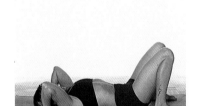

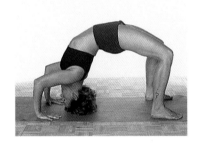

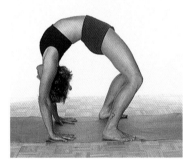

Do not strain to get into this pose; if you find it difficult, practise the pelvic lift modification. Avoid straining your back and shoulders.

DRISHTI (GAZE POINT): NOSE

Full posture:

1. Press your palms beside your ears, with your fingertips tucked under your shoulders. Keep your feet parallel and grounded (1).

2. Inhale, raise the hips, press through the palms of your hands and rest the crown of your head on the floor (2). You may need to stop at this stage.

3. If you can, lift your head and straighten your arms, opening the top of your chest in a deep arch (3).

4. Breathe deeply into your spine and seal the lower locks.

5. Take five Ujjayi breaths.

6. Repeat this posture three times. If possible, rest the crown of your head on the mat between each full lift.

7. Gently release the posture as you exhale.

mod 1   **mod 2**   **mod 3**

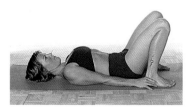

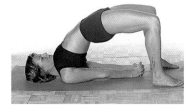

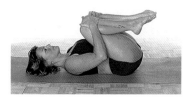

MODIFICATION:

This pelvic lift is ideal for beginners.

1. Lie semi-supine, with your spine lengthened and your neck released **(mod 1)**.

2. Tuck your heels close into your sitting bones, keeping your feet parallel. Anchor down the big toe joints and spread the balls of the feet wide. The alignment of the feet is essential.

3. Inhaling, lift your hips to the sky, raising the pelvis as high as you can, avoiding strain in the lumbar region (lower back). Clasp your hands under your body, keeping your arms straight, creating a deep lift in your thoracic spine and an opening in your shoulders, stretching the muscles in your neck **(mod 2)**.

4. Relax your face and keep your brow smooth, i.e. don't frown!

5. Take five Ujjayi breaths.

6. Exhale and uncurl your spine like a fern, pressing the lower part of your spine into the mat before your pelvis. Hug your thighs into the wall of your abdomen to counterpose **(mod 3)**.

7. Repeat this posture three times.

BENEFITS

The Upward Facing Bow is an intense stretch through the spine and the front body, massaging and toning the abdominal organs. Healthy blood nourishes the shoulders and neck and the heart is open.

PASCHIMOTTANASANA – TUNING THE WEST POSTURE

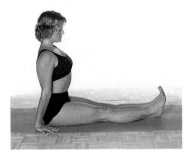 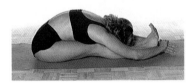 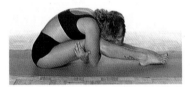

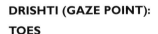

DRISHTI (GAZE POINT): TOES

1. Roll up to a sitting position and assume Dandasana, the seated Staff pose. Lift away the flesh of your buttocks, stretch out your legs, pressing the backs of your knees down by flexing your feet up (**1**).

2. Lengthen your spine, pushing your thoracic spine between your shoulderblades. Roll back your shoulders and lift your chest, sealing the abdominal wall inwards.

3. Lift your root lock.

4. Inhale, open your chest and shoulders.

5. Exhale, fold your upper body over your legs into a forward bend to ease out the lower back and counterpose the back bend. Catch your feet with your hands and lift your front ribs away from your pelvis (**2**). Do not force the upper part of your body or tighten your shoulders. With practice, the lower back will release. (If necessary, bend your knees and press your abdomen onto your thighs, so as not to strain the lower back, and keep the spine lengthened.)

6. Expand your breathing into your side-ribs. Take 20 Ujjayi breaths.

7. Make your breathing even deeper now, as you move into the final phase of the practice.

8. Inhale, look up and open your heart.

9. Exhale and lie down on the mat in

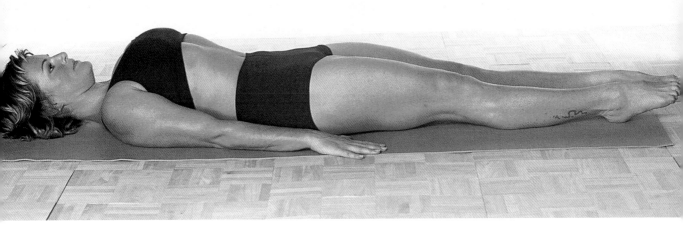

Savasana, the Corpse pose.

10. Take five Ujjayi breaths.

MODIFICATION

If you cannot reach your hands round your feet, just clasp them round your knees instead **(mod)**.

SAVASANA (CORPSE POSE)

1. Lie flat on your mat and realign your body either side of your spine.

2. Open your shoulders, broaden your chest across the top, widen your pelvis and straighten your legs.

3. Make your arms straight, and press your palms down beside your hips.

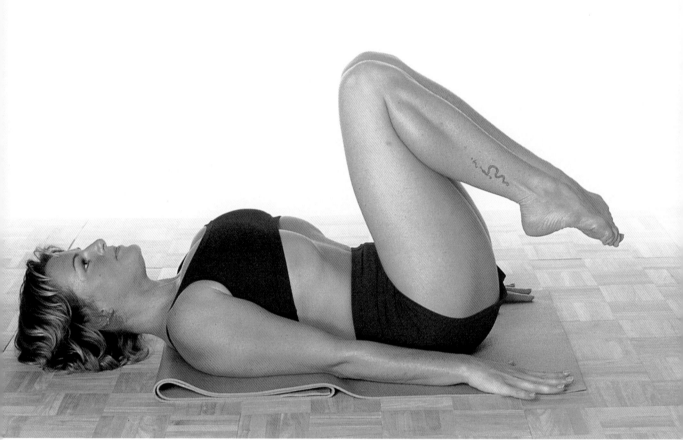

SALAMBA SARVANGASANA – SUPPORT ALL LIMBS POSTURE – THE SHOULDERSTAND CYCLE

DRISHTI (GAZE POINT): NOSE

CAUTION: Do not practise this cycle if you are pregnant (work with a specialist teacher), or have eye, ear, neck or lumbar problems, or suffer from high blood pressure or have had recent surgery on your eyes or ears.

Fold your mat into four layers to provide a padded support for your shoulders, neck and upper back. It is beneficial if the head is lower than the shoulders to keep freedom in the neck and avoid pressure on the cervical spine (the neck vertebrae). Beginners must learn the following two inversions with an experienced teacher.

1. From Savasana, the Corpse pose, inhale and bend your knees, tucking them into your abdomen, which is drawn inward **(1)**.

2. Swing your legs and pelvis up, raising your hips and cupping your lower back with both hands. Keep breathing fully and freely **(2)**.

3. As you breathe, lift your trunk higher, checking there is no strain on the neck Do not look sideways!

4. Bring your spine to a vertical position, walking your hands higher up your back towards your thoracic

and shoulders. Bend your knees and place your feet on the wall, parallel and hip-width apart.

2. Inhale and raise your pelvis, drawing your navel to your spine, lifting your pelvic floor. Cup your lower back with your hands.

3. Remain in this position and take 20 deep Ujjayi breaths.

4. Exhale and carefully lower your body down, returning to rest your legs against the wall.

5. Counterpose this posture by hugging your thighs into your abdomen, rocking in a sideways motion. Listen to your lower back. Ease it out, massaging the lumbar muscles into the mat.

BENEFITS:

Known as "the Queen of all asanas", Sarvangasana harmonizes all the bodily systems, balancing particularly the endocrine (hormonal) system and stimulating the thyroid gland situated in the throat. Healthy blood flows to the head, neck and upper torso, resting the heart and brain and easing headaches. The shoulderstand also helps to build immunity to colds and sore throats. Venous blood returns to the heart, draining the legs and abdominal organs, thus freeing the body of toxins. Constipation and bladder problems are relieved, while digestion is strengthened and the inner organs are purified.

2

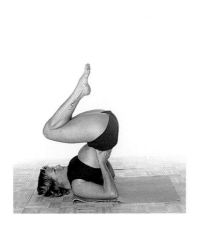

3

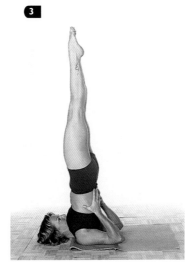

spine, but keep supporting your back firmly.

5. Aim to touch your chest to your chin, emphasizing Jalandhara bandha, the throat lock which stretches and controls the breath **(3)**.

6. Support your body on your shoulders and upper arms. Never put any strain on the cervical part of your spine (the neck).

7. Point your toes and straighten your legs, pressing the inner seams of your legs together. Your elbows should be in line with your shoul-

ders, not splayed open.

8. Take 30 deep Ujjayi breaths.

MODIFICATION:

This is an alternative to the shoulderstand for beginners and those with cervical (neck) or lumbar (lower back) problems. Lie with your hips touching the base of the wall and your legs raised up it. Relax!

1. Make sure you have a padded mat (see the introduction to the full posture opposite) beneath your spine

mod

I

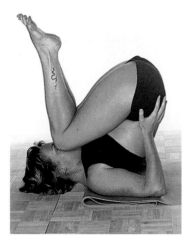

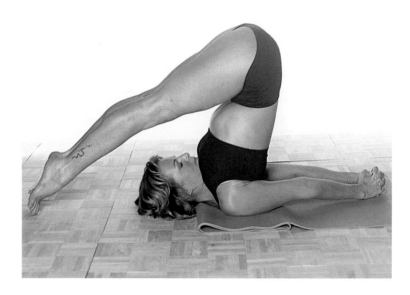

HALASANA – PLOUGH POSTURE

DRISHTI (GAZE POINT): NOSE

1. From the shoulderstand, exhale, and keeping your legs strong and straight, with the inner seams pressed together, lower them over your head so that the tips of your toes touch the mat behind your head.
2. Keep lifting your sitting bones, sealing your navel towards your spine. If your back feels stable, and your neck free, place your arms on the floor behind you, makng a "z" shape with your body.
3. Clasp your hands, squeezing your shoulderblades together to create a deeper lift upwards, out of the shoulders **(I)**.
4. Stretch through your arms, spine and legs. Don't be passive in the pose. Lift and lengthen.
5. Take 10 Ujjayi breaths.

MODIFICATION:

Drop your knees to rest on your brow. Do not force or strain your-self. Keep your back supported with your hands until you are ready to explore further asanas. Hollow your lower belly and listen to the ebb and flow of your breathing **(mod)**.

BENEFITS:

The benefits of this posture are similar to those gained from practising Sarvangasana, with the bonus that it also exercises the abdominal muscles. Forward bending nourishes the spine, opens the shoulders and purifies the intestines.

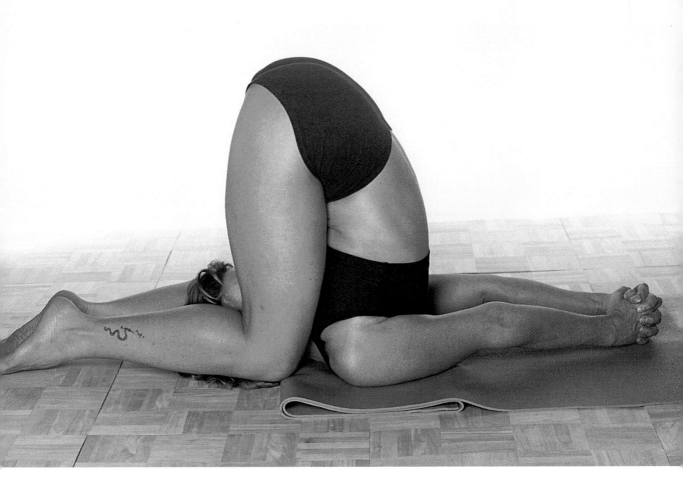

KARNAPIDASANA – EAR PRESSURE POSTURE

DRISHTI (GAZE POINT): NOSE

1. From Halasana, exhale and bend your knees, aiming to squeeze your ears with your knees.
2. Bring your inner heels and big toes to meet, and point your toes.
3. Continue to draw in the wall of your abdomen. Sealing off your hearing, you are now practising pratyahara, the fifth limb of yoga, i.e. withdrawal of the senses.
4. Take 10 Ujjayi breaths.

BENEFITS:

This pose allows you to rest your heart, back and legs. It also sharpens hearing and the deep stretch nourishes the spine and tones the waist.

You should practise the next three asanas only under the guidance of a teacher. If that is not possible, omit them and close the sequence, uncurling your spine on the mat. Then move on to Matyasana (the Fish posture – see page 136).

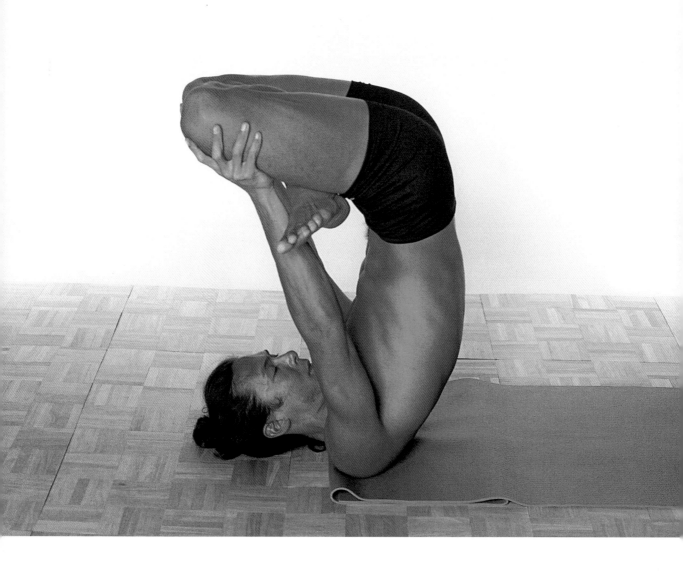

URDHVA PADMASANA – HIGH LOTUS FLOWER

DRISHTI (GAZE POINT): NOSE

1. Inhale and lift your legs up, returning to Sarvangasana, the shoulderstand.

2. Bend your knees, crossing your right leg into a half Lotus, without forcing your knee. Then place your left foot on to your right thigh, in a full Lotus posture. Don't strain your knees.

3. Press your hands on your thighs and balance in this inverted Lotusflower posture. Cultivate Uddiyana bandha, the abdominal lift; Jalandhara bandha, the throat lock and Mula bandha, the root lock.

4. Take 10 Ujjayi breaths.

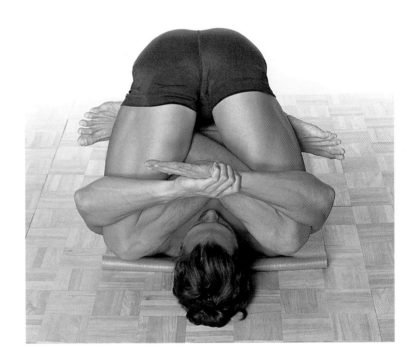

PINDASANA – EMBRYO POSTURE

DRISHTI (GAZE POINT): NOSE

1. Breathing mindfully, bring your knees to your ears, enveloping your legs with your arms to resemble an embryo. Clasp your hands, aiming to hold the wrists.
2. Listen to the breath echoing through your body.
3. Take 10 Ujjayi breaths.

MODIFICATION FOR URDHVA PADMASANA AND PINDASANA:

Practise the half Lotus by placing your right foot into a half Lotus and lower the straight left leg to the floor in the manner of Halasana. Take 10 Ujjayi breaths and change sides. This is good for loosening the hips and developing flexibility for the full Lotus posture.

BENEFITS OF URDHVA PADMASANA AND PINDASANA:

The lower abdomen and the pelvic region are purified, and the liver, spleen and stomach cleansed. The stomach and colon are massaged, so relieving constipation, and the spine is stretched beautifully.

1

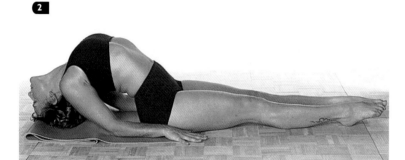

2

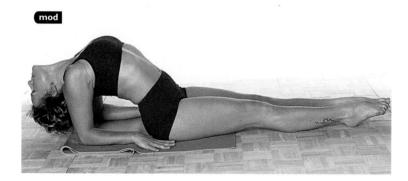

mod

advanced

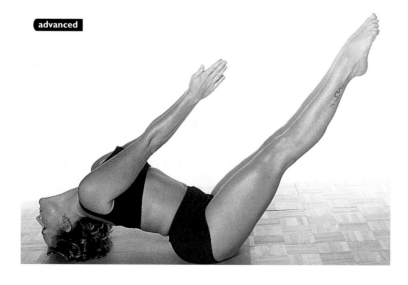

MATSYASANA – FISH POSTURE

Matsya is the God of the fishes. The creation of Hatha Yoga is traditionally associated with Goraksha Natha and his teacher Matsyendra Natha who were both born in Bengal and to whom Krishnamacharya's lineage can be traced. Matsyendra was an originator of "Nathism", which refers to the yogic adepts (nathas) who roamed the Himalayas and were considered immortal beings, enjoying both liberation (mukti) and paranormal powers. Matsyendra, meaning "lord of fish" is venerated as the deity guarding Kathmandu.

DRISHTI (GAZE POINT): NOSE

1. From Sarvangasana, the Shoulder-stand cycle, exhale and release your arms, pressing your palms into the mat.

2. Stretch your legs straight out in front of you, pressing the inner seams of your legs together **(1)**. Point your toes.

3. Inhale and lift your chest, arching your spine to release the crown of your head into the mat. **(2)** If possible, place the crown of your head on the mat. If this is too intense, lean on your elbows and let your head drop gently back **(mod)**. Use your elbows to support the lift and to open your chest. Concentrate on the centre eye, the space between your eyebrows, and relax your face.

4. Take 10 Ujjayi breaths.

ADVANCED MATSYASANA (FULL POSTURE)

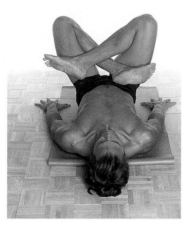

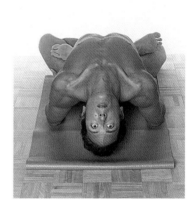

5. Advanced practitioners should aim to lift their arms up and bring their palms together like an arrow and lift their feet up at a 45-degree angle, while keeping the crown of the head on the mat **(advanced)**.

DRISHTI (GAZE POINT): THIRD EYE

Do not practise this if you have any injury to your neck.

If you are in Padmasana, the Lotus position, stay in it and gently uncurl your spine into the mat like a fern. Continue to breathe mindfully.

1. Exhale and release your spine into your mat **(1)**.

2. Inhale, arch your spine and lift your neck and chest. Open your shoulders and place the crown of your head on to the mat **(2)**.

3. To deepen the pose, catch your toes with your hands and inhale. Arch your spine higher and create openness in your heart and lungs.

4. Take 10 Ujjayi breaths,

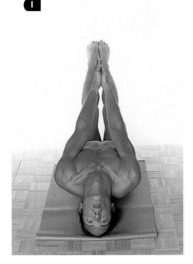

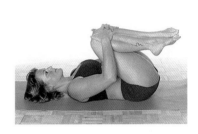

UTTANA PADASANA – EXTENDED LEG POSTURE

Don't practise this posture if you have any injury to the lumbar region. Instead, to counterpose the Fish, curl your spine by hugging your thighs into your lower back to ease out your lumbar spine.

DRISHTI (GAZE POINT): NOSE

If you are in the Lotus position, release it now to straighten your legs.

1. Inhale and lift your outstretched, straight legs to a 45-degree angle **(1)**. Harness Uddiyana bandha very strongly, utilizing the strength in your abdominal muscles to sustain the leg lift.
2. Take 10 Ujjayi breaths.
3. You can now move into Chakorasana (the Wheel pose) and from there into Vinyasa if you wish.
4. Place the palms of your hands beside your ears and roll your legs over like a wheel.
5. Press your palms into the mat to avoid putting pressure on the back of your neck.
6. If possible, land in the Staff pose so that you can go straight into Vinyasa.

MODIFICATION:

1. Do not put any pressure on your neck. Lift the upper part of your body to lean on your elbows.
2. Inhale, lift your chest high and breathe into the bottom corners of your lungs.
3. Exhale and gently release your head back with care.

If this posture causes any pain in the neck area, counterpose it with a gentle rock on the spine, hugging your knees into your thighs **(2)**.

BENEFITS:

Matsyasana is excellent for breathing problems because it opens the chest to encourage deep breathing. It also helps to nourish the thyroid gland, liver and spine. Plus it helps to open the shoulders and strengthen the neck and back muscles.

Uttana Padasana, often called the "Speak from the heart" pose, helps to strengthen the quality of your voice, so it is excellent for singers and performers. It is written in yoga texts that it improves the ability to pronounce words correctly. (Perhaps we should introduce it in schools!)

The Sarvangasana cycle strengthens the skeletal system, purifies the blood and the nerves and stimulates digestion.

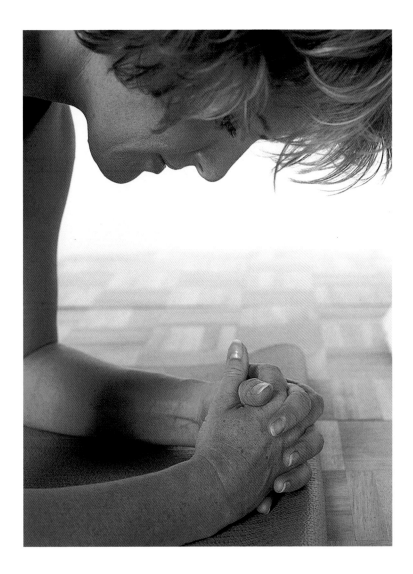

SALAMBA SIRSASANA – SUPPORT HEAD POSTURE

Don't learn this posture without the guidance of a teacher.

If you are a beginner, use a wall to help you practise it at first. Eventually, you should be able to support your body internally with the use of the bandhas and the strength of your spine, legs and arms.

DRISHTI (GAZE POINT): NOSE

1. Fold your mat in half to create a padded base. Kneel in front of the base of the mat. (Beginners should be facing a wall for support.)

2. Place your forearms on the mat and fold them at the elbows, then open your palms and clasp your hands. This forms a firm triangular base for the headstand.

3. Place the back of your head in your cupped hands, with the crown of your head touching the floor.

4. Press your weight equally through your wrists and elbows to create a firm foundation.

5. Lift your hips up, tip-toeing your feet towards your body. Do not strain your neck, but keep it long and lengthen through your spine.

6. Inhale and raise both feet up, bending your knees ([2] on page 140).

7. Establish your balance by cultivating the bandhas and concentrating on your breathing and keep your spine long and straight.

8. Straighten your legs, pressing the inner seams of them together, and pointing your toes.

9. Lift your shoulders away from your ears so as not to compress the

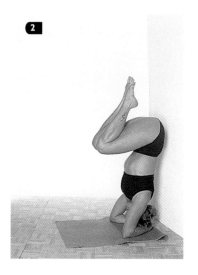

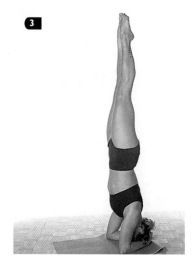

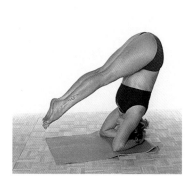

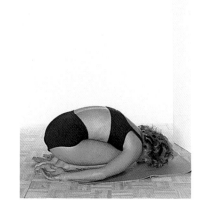

cervical spine (neck) **(3)**.

10. The back of your head, the backs of your thighs, and your spine should be in line.

11. Take 30 Ujjayi breaths, finding steadiness in the asana.

12. To come out of the posture, bend your knees into your abdomen, and as you exhale bring your legs down to the floor to a kneeling position.

ADVANCED PRACTICE:

With practice, enter and exit the posture with straight legs, hingeing from the hips as the axis of movement, using the strength of the abdomen – as in the Handstand **(4)**. Always inhale as you lift up and exhale as you lower yourself.

COUNTERPOSE
(OR RECOVERY POSTURE):

Rest and breathe in the Child's pose, i.e. kneeling and curled up, with your brow to the floor and your arms by your sides **(5)**. Relax and take 30 Ujjayi breaths.

BENEFITS:

Known as the "King" of all asanas, this produces the same benefits as the shoulderstand, soothing and balancing both body and mind. It cleanses the organs of the five senses and helps to increase your memory. This crowning posture which completes the practice is said to "raise the bindu", i.e. raise the inner light of illumination to the top chakra (see Chapter 8).

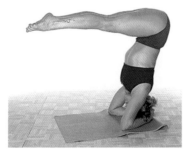

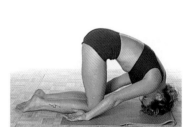

URDHVA DANDASANA – UPSTAFF POSTURE

This posture is optional and should be attempted only by advanced practitioners.

DRISHTI (GAZE POINT):

1. From Salamba Sirsasana: exhale and lower your straight legs to a 90-degree angle, harnessing the bandhas. Keep your legs really straight, and move your hips back to balance your weight evenly (**1**).
2. Take five Ujjayi breaths, then raise your legs.

ADVANCED PRACTICE:

1. Additionally, aim to lift your head 2in off the floor, supporting the weight of your body entirely on your forearms.
2. Take 10 Ujjayi breaths.

MODIFICATION:

As an alternative to the Headstand, practise the Raised Child's pose. From the Child's pose, lift your hips, rolling up on to the crown of the head (**mod**). Take 10 Ujjayi breaths.

BENEFITS:

The inversion rests the abdomen and colon, relieving constipation; the spine is stretched, and the stomach massaged. The Raised Child's pose alleviates tension in the head and neck.

FINAL BREATHING SEQUENCE

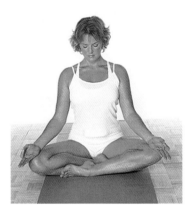

BADDHA PADMASANA – BOUND LOTUS FLOWER POSTURE

This is an advanced posture.

DRISHTI (GAZE POINT): NOSE

1. From Dandasana, the Seated Staff pose, move into Padmasana, the Lotus pose. Bend your right leg, press your shinbone to your thigh bone and draw your knee back so that you can feel the movement initi-ated from your hip rotation. Do not strain your knee.

2. Rotate in your hip joint, to bring your right foot on to your left thigh. Then do the same on the left side, lifting the left foot carefully on to the right thigh. **(1)**

3. (Advanced practitioners only) To bind the pose, reach your arms behind your back and clasp your right big toe with your right hand and your left big toe with your left hand.

MODIFICATION:

If you cannot assume the Lotus pos-ture, draw your right heel into the perineum, and place your left heel in front of the right foot **(mod)**. (This is Siddhasana, the Perfect posture.)

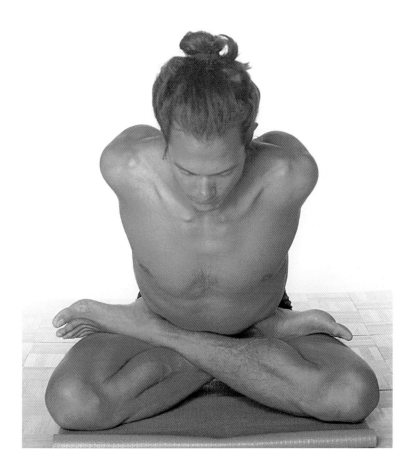

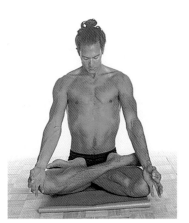

YOGA MUDRA – SEALED YOGA POSTURE

DRISHTI (GAZE POINT): THIRD EYE

1. Exhale and lean forwards, with your chin towards the floor **(1)**.
2. Hollow your lower belly to cultivate Uddiyana bandha and take 10 Ujjayi breaths. (If possible, your big toes should be clasped, or bound.)

PADMASANA – LOTUS

DRISHTI (GAZE POINT): NOSE

1. Inhaling, return to the Lotus posture. Aim to press your heels into the sides of your lower abdomen **(2)**.
2. Take 25 Ujjayi breaths. Focus. Lower your eyelids, relax your brow and soften your mind.

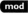

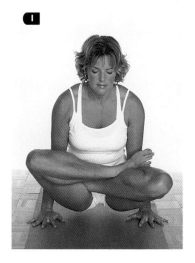

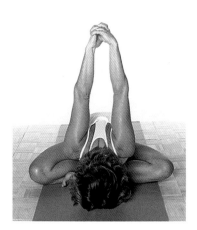

TOLASANA – PAIR OF SCALES POSTURE

DRISHTI (GAZE POINT): NOSE

1. Place your hands on the floor either side of your thighs. Use the strength of your arms and the lower bandhas to lift your body off the floor, holding your knees as high as possible **(1)**. Keep your chin tucked down a little to maintain length through the back of your neck.

2. Take 25 Ujjayi breaths deeply and slowly.

3. Move into a final Vinyasa. Advanced practitioners should aim to jump back into the final Vinyasa.

MODIFICATION:

This is a modified breathing sequence.

1. Sitting in Siddhasana, clasp your hands behind your back to open your chest and heart.

2. Inhale, lift your chest and look up.

3. Exhale, and fold your head and torso forwards towards the floor, aiming to touch your brow to the floor **(mod)**.

4. Take 10 Ujjayi breaths.

5. Inhale and return to a seated posture, keeping your spine as straight as possible and your shoulders wide.

6. Take 25 Ujjayi breaths.

BENEFITS:

This posture is the classic asana for practising the higher limbs of yoga, dharana and dhyana (concentration and meditation). The Lotus posture keeps the mind alert and brings flexibility to the knees, ankles and hips. It purifies the liver, colon and spleen, and helps to straighten the spine. Blood flows to the lumbar region and pelvis.

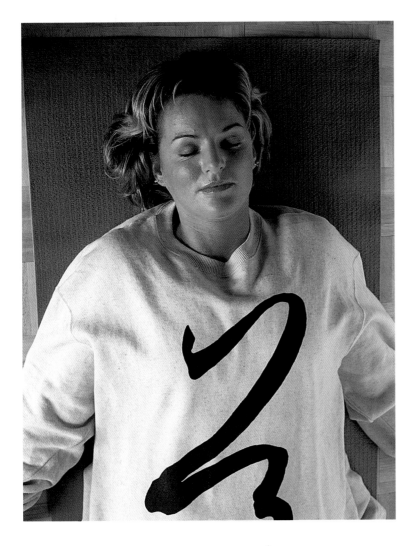

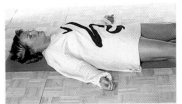

FINAL SAVASANA – CORPSE POSE.

1. Gently bring your body to the floor, lengthening your spine as you lie down. Release the lumbar spine by moving your tailbone away from the crown of your head, and lower your chin towards your chest to release the neck muscles.

2. Bring your arms down by your sides, widening the space between your shoulderblades, and press your shoulders deep into the mat, pushing them away from your ears.

3. Let your palms turn upwards, fingertips curling in, and let your toes fall outwards.

4. Close your eyes and feel your shoulders and pelvis become heavy as your body drops like a stone into the mat. Let go of your limbs, allowing your muscles to relax, and creating a sense of internal space. Drop your breath back down into your lower abdomen as you release the locks and the controlled breathing. It is very important now to relax the bandhas completely, and the Ujjayi breathing, softening the lower belly and feeling your navel rise with every inhalation and fall with every exhalation.

5. Relax your face, soften your brain and keep your body still in order to absorb the practice.

This should take a minimum of 10 minutes.

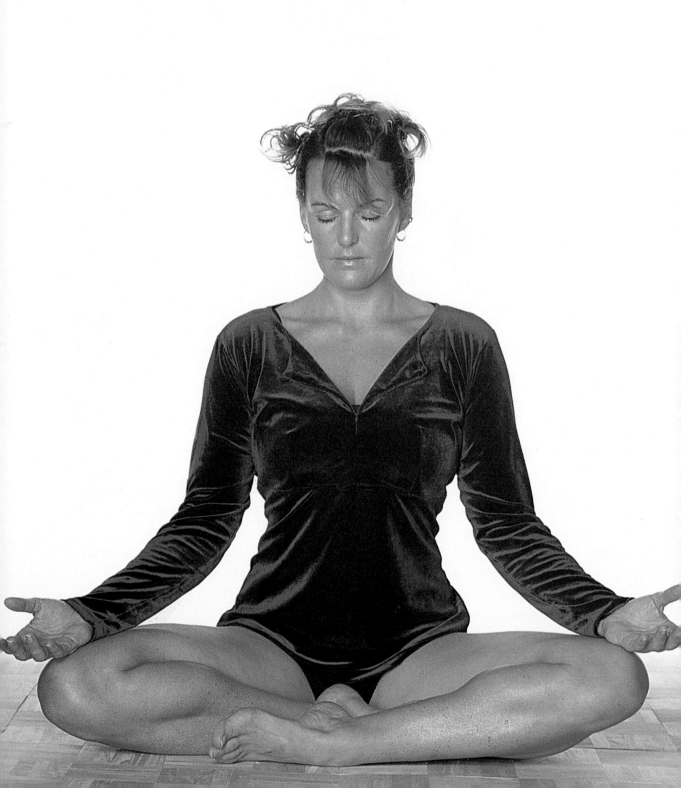

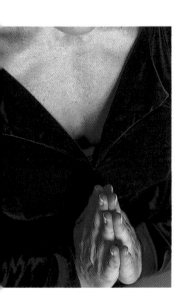

7

THE IMPORTANCE OF RELAXATION - YOGA NIDRA (YOGIC SLEEP)

This chapter emphasizes the importance of relaxation in order to absorb the benefits of the dynamic, cleansing practice of Astanga Vinyasa Yoga (Eight-limbs breath-synchronized movement and balance).

Increased levels of fitness and health are clear benefits of this form of yoga. Ultimately, the practice is aimed at bringing about a state of balance to all areas of one's life, and the stillness of mind is the essence.

Relaxation is best practised after the asanas, but Yoga Nidra can be practised separately, after work or before going to sleep, to shift into a different mind-set and to de-stress at the end of your day.

We have come again to that knee of seacoast no ocean can reach.

Tie together all human intellects, they won't stretch to here.

The sky bares its neck so beautifully, but gets no kiss.

Only a taste.

This is the food that everyone wants, wandering the wilderness.

"Please give us your manna and quail."

We're here again with the beloved.

RUMI, THIRTEENTH-CENTURY SUFI MYSTIC.

RESTORING BALANCE

The majority of postures in the Primary Series focus on the massage and detoxification of the abdominal organs, particularly the intestines.

Following the intensely cleansing practice of Astanga Yoga, it is fundamental to learn the art of relaxation, of letting go, for the release of tension restores balance to the bodily processes, and is the secret of transformation.

The most effective way to remove tension is firstly to exaggerate it. Physical and mental relaxation is brought about by the systematic contraction and relaxation of muscles all over the body.

Many of us think we are relaxing by sipping a piña colada or sitting in front of the TV with a coffee, but this is sensory diversion rather than relaxation, and many of us go to sleep with unresolved tensions. Just as we need to process and digest food, we need to process and digest emotions and experiences. Otherwise we accumulate mental and emotional, as well as physical, toxins, leading to psychosomatic, i.e mind/body related, disease.

Yoga philosophy defines three types of tension which create disease:

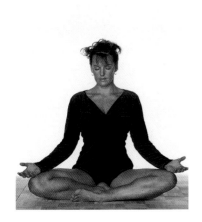

> The only devils in this
> world are those running
> around in our own hearts,
> and that is where all our
> battles ought to be fought.
>
> **GANDHI**

MUSCULAR:

This affects the nervous system, and causes endocrine (hormonal) imbalances.

EMOTIONAL:

Stemming from conflicting dualities, i.e, love/hate, success/failure, happiness/unhappiness, and unexpressed emotions.

MENTAL:

Brought about by excessive mental activities, too much thinking!

Yoga Nidra, described by the Bihar School of Yoga in Mungar in India as sleep with a trace of awareness, is a science of relaxation, offering techniques to drop the conscious mind and dive deep into the realms of the subconscious to release tensions and establish harmony in all aspects of our being. It involves the practice of sense-withdrawal, pratyahara, the fifth limb of yoga.

It is believed that in order for there to be balanced functioning, we need harmony between the upper brain (consciousness) and the lower brain (the seat of the subconscious). Conflict between the two creates a dichotomy in human nature. There also needs to be balance between the left and right hemispheres of the brain.

Yoga Nidra integrates the logical left side of the brain, which is linear and worldly, with the non-logical right side, wherein our creativity and inspiration lie. This is the part which inspires artists and musicians, often leading them into a world of their own. For example, Van Gogh painted as if he was in a dream state, Mozart composed in his sleep, Goethe solved problems and Einstein accelerated his awareness by exploring the inner realms of the mind.

Jung believed that a balanced, integrated person must access the unconscious mind, the shadow – the part which is not seen – and bring it to light as a way of knowing ourselves and understanding our motivations. He asserted that the unconscious mind is the base of man's drives, of his or her normal and abnormal behaviour.

In the state of Yoga Nidra, the brains focused effortlessly. Positive thoughts can replace negative motivations, intuition can be developed, samskaras lifted and discoveries made.

THE TOOLS OF YOGA NIDRA

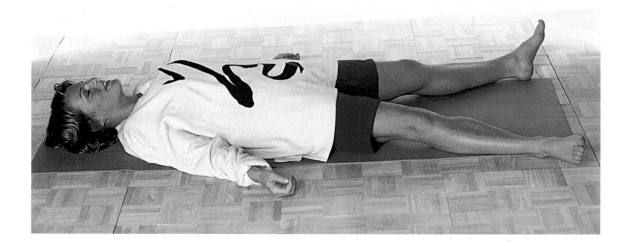

SANKALPA:

A positive statement to focus one's life in a particular direction. It is sown like a seed in the bed of the subconscious mind where it is nurtured.

ROTATION OF CONSCIOUSNESS:

A systematic exercise to rotate the mind on different body parts, cultivating awareness.

BREATHING AWARENESS:

Cellular breathing cleanses, calms and promotes relaxation and concentration.

FEELINGS AND SENSATIONS:

The pairing of feelings (hot and cold etc.) balances the left and right sides of the brain which helps to bring about emotional balance.

VISUALIZATION/GUIDED IMAGERY:

Mental relaxation and self-awareness is developed through images and symbols.

CLOSE:

A peaceful image leading to our positive resolve (sankalpa) before gently awakening.

PREPARATIONS

1. The ideal time to practise is early morning or evening, in semi-darkness.
2. Practise in Savasana, ideally after asana practice.
3. Beginners should learn with a qualified teacher.
4. Once learnt, you can practise from a tape.
5. Wear warm comfortable clothing. Be snug!

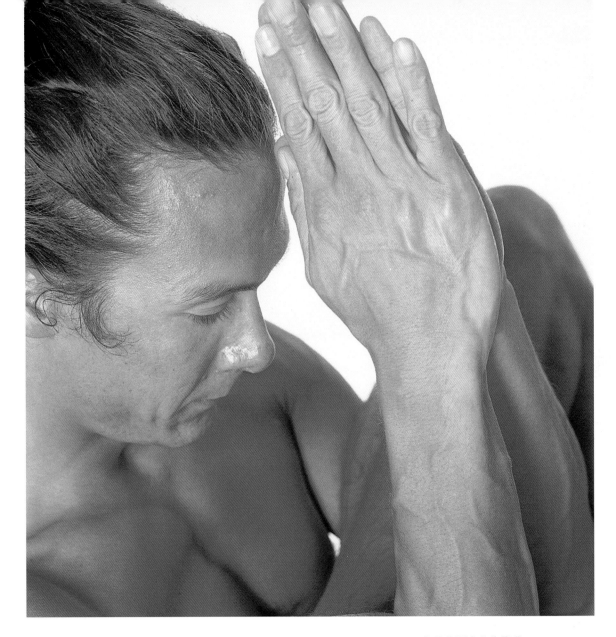

Read slowly the following guided practice, which is an example of Yoga Nidra as taught by the Bihar School of Yoga. Enter into the experience and feel the effects as you read.

RELAXATION

Lie on the floor, in the Savasana pose (see page 145) and keep warm. Relax your whole body, checking that your spine is straight and your head and neck are released. Let your limbs fall open either side of your spine, while your toes fall outwards and your palms face upwards.

Close your eyes, allowing them to soften, and turn your attention inwards.

Take a deep, full breath, and as you exhale, allow your body to drop deep into the mat.

Become aware of your whole body , and notice any sensations.

Feel the weight of your body releasing into the floor with every exhalation.

Pause

SANKALPA - AFFIRMATION

As you relax, allow a short, positive statement to form in your mind.

Pause

Gently repeat it to yourself, three times, with conviction.

Pause

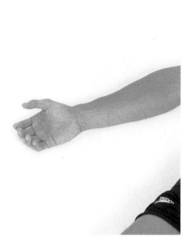
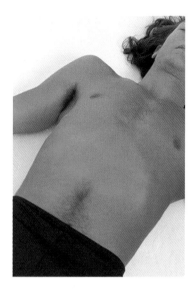
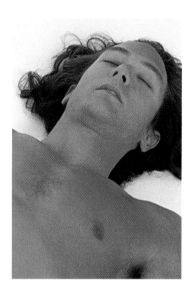

BODY SCAN - DROPPING THE MIND INTO THE BODY

As you relax, bring your awareness directly to the following parts of the body, pausing between each and scanning them in your mind:

Bring your awareness into the palm of your right hand... the back of the hand... the wrist... the forearm... elbow... the upper arm... the right shoulder... the right waist... the right side of your pelvis... the top of the right leg... the knee... the calf... the right ankle... the top of the right foot... the sole of the right foot... the toes...

Now repeat the above instructions on the left-hand side, slowly, beginning with the palm of the left hand. (Say them to yourself.)

Pause

Bring your awareness into the back of your body lying on the floor. Become aware of your right shoulderblade... the left shoulderblade... the right lower back... the left lower back... the right buttock... the left buttock... relax the whole of your back into the floor...

Keep relaxed but do not fall asleep.

Now take your awareness to the crown of your head... bring your awareness into your skull... the brow... the right eye... the left eye... the right cheek... the left cheek... the right side of your face... the left side of your face... the throat... the collarbones... moving your awareness down, relax the right collarbones... the left collarbones... the right ribs... the left ribs... draw your awareness to the belly... the lower belly... the navel...

Now bring your awareness into the right leg... from the pelvis to the toe-tips... and into the left leg... from the left hip to the toe-tips... become aware of both legs together... release the length of the right arm... release the length of the left arm... release both arms together... release the whole body together... become aware of your whole body... gently relaxing on the floor...

Pause

BREATHING AWARENESS

Now listen to the sound of your breath... become aware of the ebb and flow of your breath... entering and exiting your body... with no effort... just awareness... of the breath... washing through the body...

Drop your mind into your abdomen... and become aware of the abdomen rising on the inhale... and

falling on the exhale... just this... keeping the abdomen soft... journey with the breath...

VISUALIZATION

Now release your awareness from your breathing and bring a soft focus into your mind's eye... allow the following pictures to crystallize in your imagination... feel them... taste them: a desert landscape... a forest glade... storm clouds gathering... a deserted ruin... the piercing sun... a full moon... the quiet earth... shining stars... torrential rain... a white lily... a red oak... a running stream... a full moon...

SANKALPA – POSITIVE AFFIRMATION

Now bring your awareness back to the positive statement that you formed at the beginning of the practice.

Do not fall asleep... keep aware, yet deeply relaxed.

This should be effortless.

Form the statement in your mind, and repeat it to yourself three times, clearly, with conviction.

CLOSING THE PRACTICE – GENTLE REAWAKENING

Become aware once more of your breathing. Follow the rhythm of each breath... with no effort... allowing the body to be completely still.

Become aware of your body in contact with the floor... feel the weight of your body on the floor... feel your body breathing...

Now become aware of the space around you... of the room around you... gently allow your body to expand as you breathe energy into it.

Slowly begin to move your fingertips and the tips of your toes. Don't rush. Take your time, awakening very slowly...

Begin to stretch now from deep inside your spine... Begin to yawn into your whole body, as if awakening from a deep replenishing sleep.

When you are ready, roll on to your right-hand side, resting as long as you need to before coming up to a sitting position.

Take your time to stretch and recover.

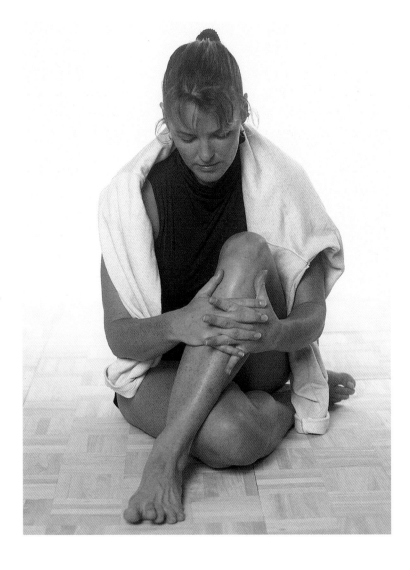

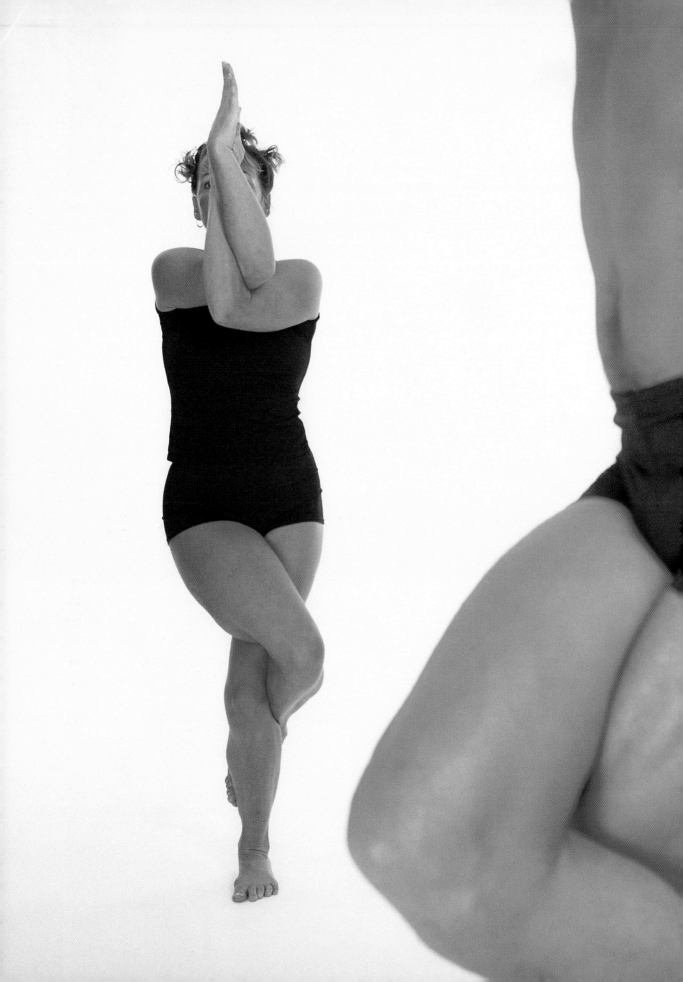

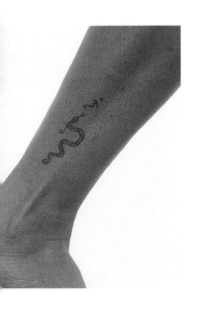

8

RAISING THE BINDU

When the body is cleansed and strengthened through the practice of asana and pranayama, an ascending pathway to awakening our inner energy begins through the eight limbs. It is as if we were removing the muddy layers which colour our perception and we become stronger, not just on a physical level but a spiritual one too, as a greater clarity develops.

This chapter briefly introduces the yogic view of the subtle energy body, explaining how it works and what it comprises.

AWAKENING THE INNER ENERGY

Our bodies are governed by the central nervous system, and the endocrine system which secretes hormones. In yoga, we move from the gross, manifest body to the subtle, metaphysical body, i.e. from the seen to the unseen. Those who practise yoga perceive that there is a parallel body in existence within ourselves, a subtle nervous system – akin to the meridians and chi of acupuncture and shiatsu – which is composed of nadis and chakras.

NADIS

The Sanskrit root meaning of nad is movement, and nadi means stream. Nadis are subtle energy channels, like threads which carry prana (life-force) throughout the body.

Similar to blood vessels, there are 72,000 nadis, the key channel being the susumna, which runs through the centre of the spine. Interweaving around the susumna channel like a Celtic knot are two subsidiary nadis called Ida and Pingala.

The Ida nadi carries the breath of the moon, which is feminine and lunar in nature, and passes through the left nostril. Its energy is maternal, emotional and nourishing. It is a calming breath.

The Pingala nadi carries the breath of the sun, which is masculine and solar in nature, and passes through the right nostril. Its energy is dynamic, vital, rational and cleansing like fire.

These two energies relate to the concept of Hatha yoga as a system of balancing the sun and moon aspects of ourselves (see page 10), in physical terms the left and the right sides of the body/mind.

Through asana and pranayama practice, the nadis are purified, and energy (prana) is able to flow through the clean channels without hindrance.

CHAKRAS

The chakras are seven energy centres situated along the spine and they are like switches. The Bihar School of Yoga in Mungar, India, describes them as "whirling vortexes of energy which exist in the etheric body of man linking points between the body and mind".

The chakras are placed at the junctions where the main nadis converge in their Celtic knot as they weave up the susumna channel through the spine and these intersections are considered to be points where the mind and the body touch.

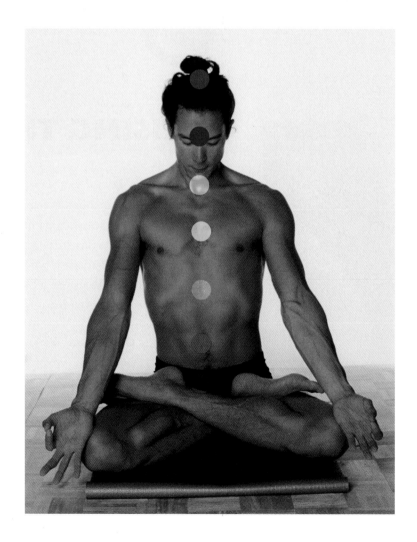

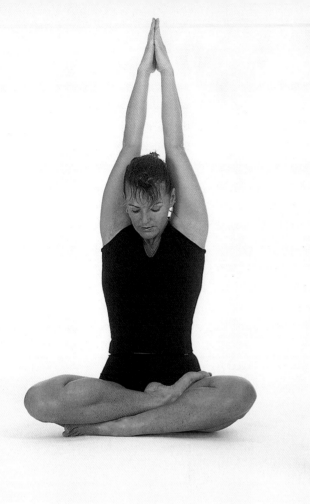

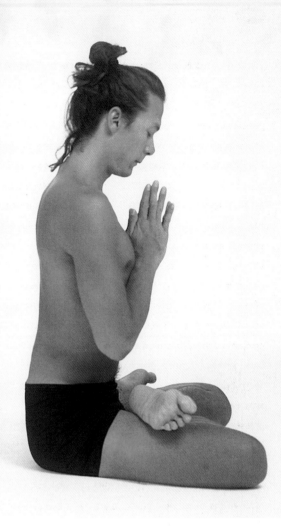

The spine is symbolized by a lotus plant with roots at its base and energy flowing upward through its sanguine stem to flower in the brain.

The chakras do not relate directly to physical organs because they function at a subtle level and cannot be seen. However they are influential, because their flowering helps to realize different aspects of one's being.

KUNDALINI – SPIRITUAL ENERGY

In yogic philosophy, Kundalini is perceived as the divine spiritual energy latent in all beings, symbolized by a coiled up snake sleeping at the base of the spine above the kanda (or bulbous root) near the navel, where the nadis unite and separate.

Kundal means coiled, and while coiled and sleeping, kundalini energy supports all life. But when awakened, she rises up the spine through the susumna, raising awareness from the lower to the higher self, spiritualizing consciousness. Carl Jung describes the impact of awakening this energy in his psychological commentary on kundalini yoga as follows: "When you succeed in awakening the kundalini so that is starts to move out of its mere potentiality, you necessarily experience a world which is totally different from our world.

"It is a world of eternity..."

As she rises through the spine towards the brain, kundalini touches each of the chakras. A vast subject of study, awareness of the chakras and focusing on them through visualization and concentration can deepen the practice of yoga. Just as Patanjali's eight limbs of yoga offer an ascending pathway (sadhana) towards integration and balance, the chakras describe seven centres in the body which symbolize a journey from the lower self to the higher self, from gross, physical reality to the subtle, transcendent reality. Each chakra provides tools to self-awareness, and can help us find our sense of place in the world.

The three lower chakras are:

MULADHARA CHAKRA

Mula means root or source and adhara means vital part. Situated at the root of the spine, the perineal and cervix area, muladhara corresponds to the organs of regeneration. The element of this chakra is earth, and it relates to our basic survival instincts, the need for security, food and shelter. It is symbolic of the earth element – of grasping the earth as one fights for survival. The colour associated with it is red.

Muladhara chakra is the meeting place of the three main nadis –Yukta Triveni, meaning three streams.

SWADISTHANA CHAKRA

Swa means one's own, interpreted as vital force or soul, and adisthana means abode or seat. This chakra, the "abode of one's own", is situated at the tip of the coccyx, and is associated with seeking personal pleasures and, while similar to Muladhara, is more concerned with appreciating things from the perspective of relationships, sensuality, friends and procreation. The Bihar School of Yoga suggests that most people in the world today predominantly function at this chakra level, seeking a connection between themselves and others. It is associated with the element of water and the colour orange.

MANIPURA CHAKRA

Meaning city of gems, the third chakra is situated in the solar plexus, the sun centre between the navel and the heart. Known as the fire centre and represented by the colour yellow, Manipura embodies· self-assertion and personal power, where one seeks to manipulate the world and gain success. The development of the ego resides here, the need for recognition. The abdominal organs – the spleen, the liver and the pancreas – relate to Manipura chakra.

One might suggest that western society is predominantly driven by the three lower chakras, the more physical, earthbound ones, which are necessary for our development in the world, but there are also four higher chakras and they are:

ANAHATA CHAKRA

Meaning unstricken, this chakra is the seat of feeling (the heart), the root of all emotions, i.e. the centre of giving and receiving unconditionally. Its element is air and it is represented by the colour green. The awakening of Anahata chakra signifies a transition from external, ego-driven power in Manipura to internal, authentic power. The gateway to the higher chakras is through the heart.

VISHUDDHA CHAKRA

Meaning pure, the Vishuddha chakra corresponds to the thyroid gland in the throat. This chakra relates to the command of language; to clarity and communication and to the search for true knowledge beyond time and cultural conditioning. When the Anahata and Vishuddha chakras are open, one speaks with clarity from the heart. It relates to the element of air and is represented by the colour turquoise.

AJNA CHAKRA

Meaning 'command, the Ajna chakra is the seat of intuition, situated in the mid-brain (usually shown at the centre of the eyebrows), and relates to the pineal and pituitary glands. The pituitary gland is the main endocrine gland, while the pineal gland is concerned with sexual function.

This third eye cultivates inner vision and psychic awareness. It is said that the physical eyes witness the past and the present while the third eye reveals insight into the future. The Ajna chakra is beyond the elements and is represented by the colour magenta.

The three nadis, Yukta Triveni, converge in Ajna Chakra having arrived from Muladhara.

SAHASRARA CHAKRA

Meaning thousand-petalled lotus, the Sahasrara chakra is the crown chakra, and relates to transcendent awareness – the eighth limb of yoga. Situated just above the crown of the head, Sahasrara corresponds also to the pineal and pituitary glands deep in the seat of the brain.

Sahasrara chakra is the seat of